Tomorrow Is Not Promised

The Story Collection
2019-2023

LUCY MASON JENSEN

Copyright © 2025 by Lucy Mason Jensen
All rights reserved.

CONTENTS

SECTION 1: Me & My friends and family 1
    Introduction to – Me & My friends & family 2
    Another turn around the sun 3
    Boy Town 6
    Fishing is not just about fishing! 8
    Forever is a very long time 10
    Friends are the family we choose 12
    Happy Birthday, dear Rita! 14
    Her Anniversary 17
    Life happens 19
    Love is all that matters 22
    Motherhood is not for wimps 25
    Sister Sheryl 27
    Sisters 29
    So much love 31
    The Dump Trailer 33
    The Mehs 35
    The move to Montana 37
    The navigation of grief 39
    The New Chair 42
    The Patience Bone 44
    The spirits of Thanksgiving past 46
    Travels with Father 48
    Visiting in situ 51
    What becomes of a broken heart? 53
    Young love 55

SECTION 2: Me & The Animals 57
    Introduction to – Me & The Animals 58
    A year with foster cats 59
    Be kind to one another 61
    Destiny arrives in funny ways 63
    Find your passion 66
    Finding Bruno 69
    Having babies in your 50's 71
    Healing llama karma 73
    My pumpkin coffee table 75
    Plenty of room in rescue 77
    Sally Comes Home 80
    Sally meets Sibyl 82

Saying bye to my boy 84
Small but beautiful things. 86
The Annual English Tea Party 88
The dreams of a rescue pup 90
The Hen Palace. 93

SECTION 3: Me & The World. 95
Introduction to – Me & The World 96
A rare and crazy adventure 97
Above all else 100
Be grateful 103
Busy people 105
Grandmas gone wild. 107
Hope is springing forth. 110
How does it make you feel?. 112
Joy Seeking. 114
My first impressions 117
Nashvegas. 120
On the circuit. 123
The 48-hour blackout 126
The Atmospheric River 128
The Coronation and other important news 130
Unmasked and Unaware 132
Writing another book 135

SECTION 4: Me & Them 137
Introduction to – Me & Them 138
Tony, Mary and me 139
Bad days, a new book and sailing around the world 141
Bright Ideas 144
Competition. 146
Cowgirl on the country circuit 148
Delighted by the youth 150
Making the time for tea 152
Never too old 154
The Lost Week 156
The Waiting 158

SECTION 5: Me & It. 161
Introduction to - Me & It. 162
A week of firsts 164
Always look on the bright side 166
Covid Year 2 168
Glass half full 170

    Health and sickness during corona 172
    Hope is not canceled. 174
    International flying with covid 176
    No need to quarantine here 178
    Opening up the world 180
    Our City by the Bay. 183
    Secret Sisters. 185
    Soap and Water. 187
    Summer Travel Woes 189
    The dolphins and the swans 192
    The Lucky. 195
    The Masked Truth 197
    The new normal 199
    The nomad. 201
    The not-fun-week. 203
    You've been 20-20ed 206

SECTION 6: Just Me **209**
    Introduction to Just ME. 210
    A New Adventure. 211
    Carmel in January. 213
    Going home again 215
    Gratitude 217
    Home for the holidays 219
    Late for it all 223
    Magic. 225
    Making good memories 227
    My big birthday 229
    October is a funny old month! 231
    Our childhood memoir. 232
    Passion 235
    Regrets 237
    Rocket Man 239
    Take care of yourself. 242
    The Best Made Plans. 244
    The books that made me. 246
    The call of the sea 248
    The gammy leg 250
    The spirits of Rosie and Winston 252
    Traveling with a cold. 254
    The time for feasting. 256
    The year that was and the one to come 258
    Waving across the valley 260

A note from the author

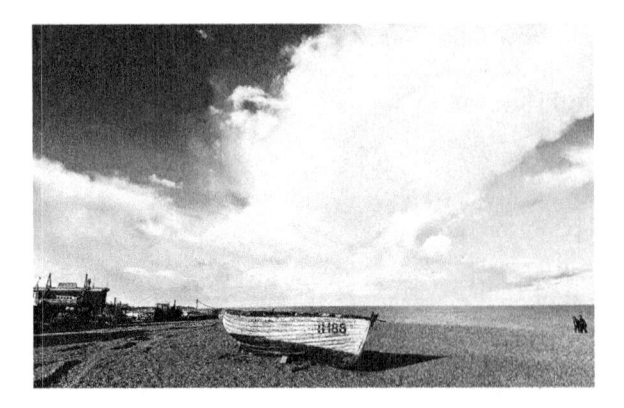

You might be wondering what the cover images of old fishing boats on a beach might have to do with tomorrow, promises, or even today or yesterday. These were the fishing boats of my childhood that are still present on the beach of my hometown in Aldeburgh on the East Coast of England. They are no longer being cared for. They are fading fast. Will they still be here tomorrow? Who knows.

Photographic evidence – old postcards, paintings, drawings of these iconic examples of yesterday's fishing industry have captured my imagination ever since I was very young, and I would watch them coming back to shore after a night at sea. I used to wonder how cold it was out there, so that the men could make a living for their family - how very lonely and sometimes scary. I do remember thinking that, although my own father seemed to spend a lot of time on a train to provide for his family, at least he wasn't alone on a boat for hours and hours at night.

These days, I go and visit the many boat sculptures that now remain on the beach, whenever I am in town – sadly many in decline – Content, Dorothy May, Viking, Two Belles, Jim Claire, Charlotte, Once More and the more uniform IH101, IH39 and so on. They are all important landmarks in my life. I hate that many are falling apart, and I do hope to somehow participate in saving at least some of them, so they can't just be images from the past but also a preserved nod to the vibrant history of the beach industry, now down to one active fishing boat that still goes out to sea daily.

In the 60's when I was born, the fisherman lived in the heart of the town and, along with the lifeboat men, (some the same people), they were the heart of the town. Now, the heart is mostly full of holiday homes and many of the local people either live up the town or have moved away entirely. The children of the old fishermen do not want any part of the industry that kept their fathers away from home many parts of most days and I clearly recall how I never wanted that for my family either! Like so many other industries, fishing is no longer, mostly, a local town trade.

Tomorrow is not promised, and change is inevitable in all aspects of life; but I do think some monuments should be preserved for the tomorrows many of us won't get to see. And that is why I chose to feature many of my beloved fishing boats inside my book. They are old friends to many and need to be revered accordingly.

Be a part of the change you wish to see.

I pledge a donation from every book sold towards the ultimate preservation of these iconic works of art or, at least, a nod to the nautical past of this divine Coast.

lucymasonjensen@gmail.com

Introduction to – Tomorrow is not promised

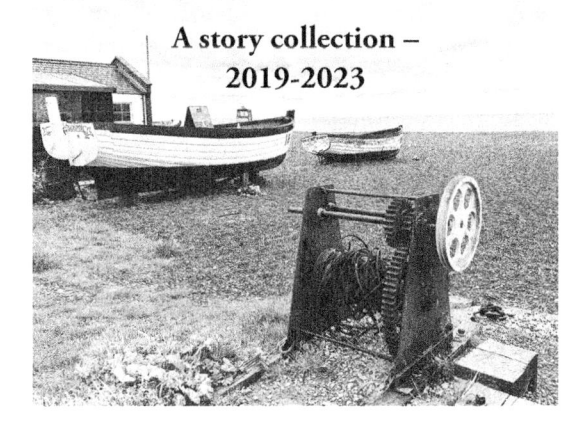

A story collection – 2019-2023

And here it is – another compilation of my stories from the local papers, formerly the Soledad Bee, The Greenfield Tribune, the Gonzales Times and the King City Rustler and now the Salinas Valley Tribune!

The way time flies I forget how many stories I write a year, how much ground I can cover in my small, sometimes extended world. "It's probably time for another compilation of stories!" Father reminds me. Bless that nonagenarian. And yes, it's been, what, 5-6 years since my last collection? It does give me great satisfaction to put all the colorful episodes into one place, as it were. Like a photo album, they do belong together as much as you can make it happen, even just as a bit of a non-chronological, wacky and always messy road map. Just like my life.

And, looking in the rearview mirror, what years have we had! Once in a lifetime kind of years! Reading back – and hopefully correctly editing as I go – I recall so clearly the January of 2020, when my friend Carey and I were in a hotel elevator in downtown San Francisco. All around us, Asian school girls in dark blue school uniforms were sporting masks. We thought they were being so weird. Move stage swiftly 2 months forward and we are all wearing masks and being quarantined to our respective bubbles in our houses. It was so unthinkable. New language evolved during that time – we were all being socially distanced and seeking high and low for coveted toilet paper and antiseptic wipes, while learning the joys of online shopping, distance learning and Zoom meetings. Horror stories still resonate in the memory bank of makeshift morgues in refrigerated trailers outside of packed hospitals. Those were some scary days.

And then the vaccine was founded in record time – marvelous - and we were so ready to get back to life and to living; but the shutdown of the world took a lot longer to reverse than it did to close down, and those were some very interesting times as well. Some of my most frustrating travels took place during the months after the actual pandemic, (with many of us having received our first vaccination), when it seemed as if the world had opened up to us travelers, but then it really hadn't. I learned a lot of patience during those days. Patience, I had perhaps accumulated from trying to travel home to see my people and being thwarted at every turn for about 18 months. I think I likely still have some travel credits floating around someplace from those dark days. In all the years I have traveled back and forth, I do not recall ever feeling so far away from my roots as I did during those peculiar months.

I remember being so worried about my daughter, an essential worker, a nurse no less, and so fearful of the virus that killed so many. Fears increased for my husband as he underwent critical heart surgery in a hospital I couldn't visit. During those difficult days that he was in intensive care, I tried to ignore inside myself my knowledge of just how very vulnerable he was to this malicious virus.

On the flip side of the horror, I also recall the peace and beauty of the clear skies at home; the gorgeous images of whales and dolphins being seen once again in the canals of Venice. I remember feeling teary at the images of voices singing out of windows at certain times of the day, thanking others - our essential workers no less - for their hard work in the line of duty. I felt as if we were witnessing the re-emergence of human priorities in some cases. The return of thoughts and lives to home, family, love – the fundamentals of a good life from what can sometimes be a trite and impatient world.

Thanks to my readers and staff of the South County Newspapers/Salinas Valley Tribune/Soledad Bee – who often remind me why I make my column deadline a weekly priority (or mostly weekly!) I enjoy writing for you and sharing our universal experiences. Thanks to my family who know I love to write and who humor me anyway, even though I'm not sure that they often read my stuff.

And to my rescue ranch at Solace – come as you are, however broken – thanks for continuing to heal my heart. Total love and respect for the pure souls that you remain.

I shall hear your voices still calling me and loving me, long after the gate is closed.

Lucy

SECTION 1

Me & My friends and family

Introduction to –
Me & My friends & family

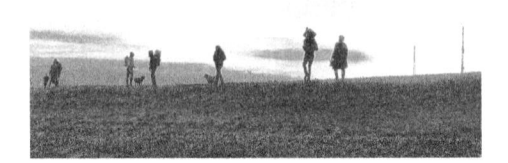

Oh, and what a big topic this is! So much to say about the many lovely people in my life and in my world! From my incredible family at home and *abroad* (which is also, oddly, my home) to my amazing friends – you know who you are and you give so much love that, sometimes, I am truly amazed at what is possible if you simply give a damn.

You learn about people when you are going through the tough stuff. When my daughter broke her back in a horrible car accident, so many people stepped forward in love and support that I was simply lifted by their caring and able to be stronger for my girl than I ever dreamed possible.

When my friend was in need of a new liver, I saw the power of love and community at its very best. We pushed and pushed and, ultimately, she received her new liver. And this is what this section of stories is about – so many things, but above all how love is really all that matters in life. And how we manage life when things look super bleak, and we cannot see our way out. That is where the friends and family come along and say, 'wow, that looks tough, how can I help?'

This section of stories is all about you – my friends and family, my people. It speaks mounds of all you folks out there that keep an eye on each other, not just me and mine, but all of us. At the end of the day, if we show up for each other, we are huge in love and light and our strength is a force to be reckoned with. And that is the way we overcome our difficulties. Together and united and loving of each other.

Thank you all – I love you more than you will ever know.

Thoughts about this section? As always, I would love to hear them. lucymasonjensen@gmail.com

Another turn around the sun

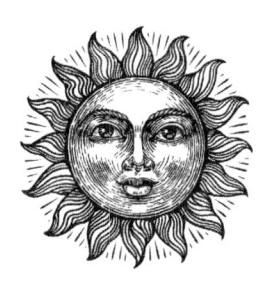

The clock ticked swiftly on, meticulously in sync with the movement of the world. The hourglass turned again and, before you knew it, I was approaching another big birthday. All birthdays are truly marvelous, honestly, another trip around the sun, a bonus chance to have more of a wonderful life on earth than you've already enjoyed. I don't struggle with aging; what's the alternative? I endeavor to embrace all the things I can still do and let go of the things I can't. It's a good mantra. My sister Rosie died at the youthful age of 48. I'm so fortunate.

But here I was back in the cottage where I was born 60 years ago with some of my very favorite people, and I do have to say that I felt quite emotional. We had cake and more cake and then some extra cake for good measure to celebrate mine and all our big birthdays. The best champagne was drunk, presents and cards opened. Enormous laughs all around. Some minutes in time you do want to frame, and this was one of them.

We went out boating on a lake that I hadn't visited since I was perhaps single digits. The lake and the rowing boats were the same. We were all a little older and a bit more cautious about falling into the two feet of water than we were years ago; but it was such a lovely outing. It's good to do one crazy thing to mark a big birthday and this was mine.

And sometimes you can have too much of a good thing; and I spent the day after my birthday mostly in bed, sleeping. Regardless of the fact it was a beautiful day, and we still had a house full of guests, I spent the day on a time out. I canceled everything for that evening and the next day and immediately felt better. Character is fate. I always want to do so much of everything until I can no more. We did make time to swing by Sutton Hoo, oh my goodness. Put it on your bucket list.

And then we were full speed ahead again and it was time to leave my lovely cottage on the East Coast of England, head back to London and then catch a flight to the Isle of Man where my sister and father live.

Weather on this little island in the Irish Sea can be a little – ahem – subject to change. Just when you think you have a lovely day ahead of you, here comes the rain or the storm or the wind; but I'm always impressed by how the locals just get on with life regardless. My sister and her lot go running, swimming, biking in all weathers. They don't really seem to notice weather! Just as well.

A family friend gave me a donkey for my big birthday. I was so excited. I'd always wanted my own donkey! Well, in actuality, it wasn't my very own to transport home to Solace in Cali, but Bluebell, The Donkey, was adopted by her for me at the lovely Home for Old Horses and Donkeys on the afore-mentioned island, where she will live out her lucky days as a very spoiled and beloved donkey. As a rescue person, plus a horse and donkey lover, I was so impressed with the home, the lovely green pastures and health and well-being of the animals at the forefront of everything. When we arrived, an old tram horse was being delivered to start his retirement on those lush acres. We took along a photo of Bluebell so she could be recognized from amongst her peers and a bag of carrots (not enough). I was so delighted by the adoption of my newest child that I felt quite moved. My sister adopted a lovely grey mare called Lady for a friend's daughter and we spent some money in their gift shop. Regardless of the rain, that was one of my most favorite days. Rescues the world over are to be saluted. I've said that before.

And then it was back to London town. Because of the unpredictability of the weather off the island, I always give myself an extra day before the flight home, just in case. Luckily my flight was on time and uneventful. The flight the following day, however, was canceled. And then I have the delightful prospect of a free day. I contacted my very old school friend Charis to see if we could meet up. We've had lovely get-togethers these past few years. She comes from her home in Reading and picks me up from my hotel at London Heathrow and then we travel to Windsor, which I have grown to like a lot. For those of you not in the know, Windsor is the location of one of the Royal Castles and the burial site of Queen Elizabeth II, Prince Philip, The Queen Mother and Princess Margaret, just to start off with. If you are a real history buff, you can find many, many more burial sites within those castle walls.

We were gifted with a gorgeously warm and sunny day – flip flop weather even – and coffee at the Ivy was in order before our tour. Truthfully, it was less of a tour and more of a time slot we were allocated to go through the rooms of the Castle and the very famous St. George's Chapel, most recently the site of Prince Philip and then the Queen's funerals. Because of the enormous distance her coffin traveled throughout the country before arriving at Windsor Castle, I had forgotten entirely that her burial was there. Charis and I stood obediently in a long line of people at the Chapel, not really knowing why, but looking around ourselves in awe at this hallowed ground. Once we realized that we would be passing by the family mausoleum and last resting place of the Queen, we became quite emotional. She was the only Queen we had ever known in our lifetime and here she was. The air in the Chapel was thick with somber pomp and majesty and we were both so very glad we had taken the time to pass through and pay our respects.

After the Chapel, we took a long time to go through the Reception Rooms at the Castle, rich with history, art and antiques. Gold-gilted everythings awaited us in those spectacular rooms until we could see no more. We agreed to revisit everything another day.

As we know from Lucy's birthday extravaganza, you can have too much of a good thing.

What a lovely day we enjoyed, eating lunch outside a super old pub with another friend from our way back childhood. So many things to catch up on and, as usual, it's as if we were never apart. It's been a marvelous turn around the sun, I do have to say. Thanks to all who participated in making it so very special.

(2023)

Boy Town

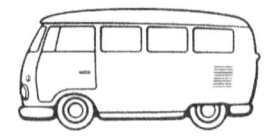

It started off as a nice offer from the husband. "He can come and stay with us for a while!" We were talking about our friend's 21-year-old son. They live in the U.K. I never thought it would happen, really didn't. "What a nice suggestion!" she responded. "Let me think on't." And then we let it go, as you do.

20-somethings the world over have a bunch of issues these days, it seems. Whether it's all the pressures of social media and looking just right, or the post-pandemic mental issues that seem to pervade the youth especially, or a combo of all of it, compounding on their undeveloped brains, I don't know. What I do know is that several of my friends with 20-something boys, (most often) are dealing with the fall-out of their mental health that takes a great strain on their families in addition, as they should be transitioning from the home to the big world outside and they don't seem to be able to do that. It's an epidemic, post pandemic, I tell you. Is there a level of entitlement mixed in there, that our generation has endorsed? I am not really qualified to say.

Anyway, time passed as she does, and my friend tells me that her son is seriously interested in coming to Cali. All the way from the UK to Cali by himself. (Yeah, believe that when I see it!) I thought to just myself. He could barely make it to college by himself; I could not conceive how this might work out.

"That's fine," I respond! (Still a non-believer.) Husband was excited, boy scout master that he is, in reality several moons ago and always at heart. And so, the seeds of *Operation Boy* were sown.

"Did boy get on the plane?" I ask. Yes, boy did. There was a little flutter right before he left, but he managed. It's as if boy knew that he needed to do this for himself and his future life. He needed to get out of his room and away from his video games, also the familiarity and comfort of his family and his home and get a taste of the world outside. "I'll email you a list," his mother said. "Oh, I thought I'd just wing it," I reply, and that was really my plan. It wasn't until I read her list that I started to feel the onus of this monumental task. I was going to have, in my care, a young man with some serious issues and the pressure was on us to try and make a difference in this young person's life in just a couple of brief weeks. I so wished I had not read that list. Despite good intentions, I am much better with animals than people.

But never fear, the scout master took charge of this young chap who was almost a mirror image of himself, truth-be-told, with matching panic attacks and social disorders. They went shopping and enjoyed cooking together. Young one learned how to make chicken enchiladas, how to master a BBQ skirt steak and manufacture some superior cherry jam, to name a few culinary experiences. He realized what an affinity he had with animals – and especially dogs – and most evenings had a dog pile right on and next to him that gave him enormous esteem. He thought about how he might get involved in animal volunteer work where he could help socialize dogs and how good he would be at that.

I saw a different side to this boy that spoke to me of how, when a person is a little off track in life, sometimes a change can be as good as a rest, as granny would say – and one trip on your lonesome can maybe alter your world for the better, if you are open to the possibilities.

"You need to help me pull the engine on Vandura," husband tells him. Knowing that boy was not a super fan of getting his hands dirty, I was curious to see how this would work out. Poor Vandura, the old VW van, was always in various states of not running. I arrive home from work to find one young chap underneath the van and one old guy sitting in the supervisory chair. Boy's hands were covered in oil. I sent a photo to his mother, and I think that tickled her heart strings just a little. Boy was stepping out of his comfort zone and trying new things. "I need to cut a hole in the wall and install that thing," husband tells him, pointing at a large box. I see the power tools coming out and rapidly make my exit. I also heard that he may have handled a (legal) firearm, but I never want to know about that stuff. It's all *boy town* to me.

For my part, I tried to teach him some domestics, picking up and cleaning around himself. This wasn't quite as successful a venture and certainly not after suppertime, but he did seem to grasp the concept that, when you live with people, you need to consciously work towards being thoughtful concerning the others and contributing to sharing a space. We discussed that topic a fair bit and the fact that his parents both work hard so that he can have a nice life and go to college. He seemed to accept that he needed to do his part and I hope that, going forward, he will.

We took him to the beach and the mountains. He enjoyed clam chowder on the wharf and the sight of an otter eating abalone on his back. We gave him a taste of Cali life that he, perhaps, hadn't imagined before and then, without even having got his bags packed to leave, he started already talking about his return visit.

I think we did pretty well with boy over the last couple of weeks. No matter I couldn't get him out of his shaggy old tennies, nor allow a glimmer of Cali sun rays to hit his white-white skin, or learn to properly clean up after himself, I think he learned some things.

And as for the husband, the old man, I was reminded that he likely missed his calling in life as a teacher or counselor; except that he didn't really miss it at all. He made a huge difference in the life of a young person these last couple of weeks and that speaks volumes about him and his abilities to effect change. Boy town is coming to a close at Solace and soon it will be just us golden oldies again. We'll see boy again out here – of that there is little doubt – and next time he'll be a pro.

(2023)

Fishing is not just about fishing!

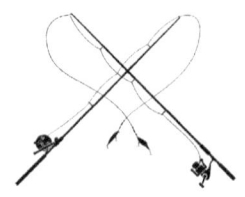

I have learned recently that fishing does not have all that much to do with catching fish. I'm sure it does in the big leagues and the commercial fisheries of the world; but in your average household that owns a couple of poles, it's more like a Sunday drive or a walk in the park. It's mind candy; a soothing of the soul, titillation of the senses. I had not known that before. My grandpa Harold was a serious fisherman. He had a whole cupboard full of poles, I do recall. He would ocean fish in the North Sea when he'd come and visit. He'd also indulge in serious fishing holidays to Scotland to catch salmon. I seem to remember he had enormous waders so he could negotiate the Scottish rivers. My granny would sit peacefully on the bank and watch and enjoy, later on, many a good fish meal, I'm sure.

When my daughter was being extricated from the wreckage of their vehicle a few short weeks ago, her pitiful voice could apparently be heard crying about the fact her fishing pole had broken. Never mind her back and most of their possessions; it was her fishing pole she was weeping over. This resonated with my dad who wanted to fix a little piece of that awful situation where he could. He sent over a gift card for her favorite fishing shop so she could replace her pole. Truthfully, the shop boasts a lot more than just fishing supplies; but it had become her new go-to emporium once she, interestingly, caught the passion of fishing from her boyfriend Aaron and then it became hers.

We did wonder how long it would take her before she got sick of being at home, safe in the cocoon of her kittens and her family. The first several days she didn't want to go anywhere that involved a vehicle. Then the 'lure' of the fishing shop gift card was dangled under her nose, and she couldn't help herself; she had to get in a car and be driven on a freeway and up to San Jose where the shop could be found. (I had suggested online shopping and got *the look*!) She and her boyfriend spent several hours in that place – up and down the aisles they went several times – and both managed to secure nice replacement poles to start moving forward from that terrible incident in their lives. She returned home absolutely beaming with delight, renewed color in her face and a sparkle in her eyes. She was now the proud owner of an ocean AND a river pole, also some new special lures.

When she was miserable and sick with pain, I had promised her I would go fishing with them once she felt better. This promise was cashed in immediately with the purchase of the new poles. We were all going to go *fishing*. My husband has always enjoyed dipping his rod, as it were, and our destination was one of his former hunting grounds, when he was a youngster with a pole and not a care in the world.

We were all packed up with bait and chairs and new rods. The only thing we forgot was our memory that Moss Landing has a very different climate to Soledad; so, jackets and blankets were a little lacking in the luggage. No matter. The fishing folk got their acts together, involving quite a lot of tying, baiting and fidgeting with rods in different places I noted, before any lines were actually cast into the water. I sat behind them with my book and my camera ready. More chit-chat, replacing of bait, (the Moss Landing fish are wiley boogers. They deliberately strip the bait off the hook and carry on, it seems), some moving of chairs, rearranging, untangling rods. I could see that fishing was a lot more than stick-pole-in-water-and-catch-something-for-dinner, as one might imagine; there was a lot of social engagement went on amongst the fishing people near the slip-slap of the brackish water and against the backdrop of herons, cormorants, pelicans and all measure of sweeping seabird. Contrary to my prior opinion, fishing was quite fun and a real pleasure for the senses. I love to be by the water, fishing or not.

I was appreciative of the porta-loo that had been thoughtfully positioned in the parking lot, also the relative shelter of the truck when the fog rolled in, as it is wont to do in that part of the world. I also shed a quiet tear or two at the sight of my back-braced kid climbing up rocks and showing us that she was still she was still beaten up, but coming back with a vengeance and, ultimately, she would be fine.

There was a lot of excitement when the senior angler hooked a large fish. The adrenalin rush was apparent, lots of cheering, whooping, photo-taking … and then the blessed thing was put back in the water. Wait, aren't you supposed to keep and cook the fish you catch? Isn't that the whole point of fishing? They looked at me as if I was nuts. (They hadn't even brought a cooler along to store said fish they might catch!) Only the *pole-less* among us apparently don't have a clue about fishing. "Mum, you can't just keep one fish!" (Even though it was a rather yummy looking skate that I have enjoyed in the past on the east coast of England.) No, I obviously didn't get it.

The next plan is to tailgate BBQ at that same place with rods in the water and skirt steak on the barby. Assuming that you are not going to catch any fish, when you go fishing, is apparently the proper outlook.

For my part, I enjoyed my first fishing trip much more than I thought I would. I was beautifully distracted by all the sea life, not to mention a few random kayakers and fledgling paddleboarders that I hoped might fall off their boards for audience value. (They didn't).

I think I shall go fishing again. When I need to just sit and be still with my lot, be happy with my hand and grateful for my blessings, I shall pack up my book and my blankets (also hats) and I shall sit in my comfy chair and enjoy the view. Who knew that there was so much more to fishing than actually catching fish!

(2021)

Forever is a very long time.

What becomes of a broken heart? In the olden days, when romantic liaisons fell apart, ladies would return home quietly to lick their wounds in private, take care of elderly relatives, or forever wear black, in mourning for the life they had wanted and lost. They would sink quietly into the shadows of life, ('Better to have loved and lost, than never to have loved at all.') Forever scarred, they might as well be widows. Nowadays, the young ladies, having fallen off the horse, get right back on it. My daughter moved down to Shell Beach to start her new life a few years ago and she made a heck of a go of it – new job, friends, apartment, boyfriend. She introduced us and all our friends to a lovely part of the world we had never known before. We thought she was all set and going to be there forever; but forever is a very long time and things fell apart with the boyfriend; she also hated her job. She could have fixed the job situation; the other not so much.

Before we knew it, she was coming home again. I remember very clearly how difficult it is to return home once you have left, especially after a good chunk of time like that. I had to do the same thing many years ago with my parents and I clearly recall how difficult it was to be back there in that house with those people. I loved them very much, but I did not want to live with them anymore. Those were tricky days – my mother asking me if I would be back in for dinner, my father asking me awkward questions about my future plans.

It was just dreadful going backwards in life like that, and I didn't stay long. But those things can change too, and, in modern times, it is very difficult for young people to live by themselves; so, returning home is not such an unusual event, if only for a little while. Home is a place to take stock, regroup, enjoy home-cooked food, do laundry without needing coins and think about what is next. It's a precious safe haven when you need it, as many of us do in life.

We rescued our daughter and her belongings from Shell Beach, dragging a cumbersome trailer behind us as we returned north again. Her dad had told her previously that he wouldn't be moving her again – and he chose to remind her of this on our journey home – and here we were. He got a mouthful from me for that. She cried all the way home and for days after. Then the light came on; she was tired of crying, and she realized that boyfriend was not really the man she had wanted him to be. She was more grieving for the life she had wanted to have, than the one she actually did. She had also adored her apartment near the water. I told her that was just geography; in time, she could recreate that.

She went on to reconnect with old friends and do some fun things. The two of us went for a run around the Bay and ate clam chowder on the wharf. She got her old job back and caught up on her sleep. These were not the days she had planned for herself, but these were the ones she needed, apparently. She helped her Mum out with poor old sick dad and started to clean out the closets and clear cabinets in the home. It started to appear that everything does happen for a reason. She had not planned on returning to her childhood house – we had not known she was going to need to; but here she was; and we were ultimately so very happy to have her back with us, diluting the difficult times we were having all by ourselves and adding an extra layer of nursing care and ability to the mix. We needed help, and she needed the port in the storm – and what a wonderfully symbiotic combination that can be, when the time is right.

What becomes of a broken heart in modern times is that you return home to heal. You find your peaceful place with the ones that truly love you and you take the time you need to come back, to rebuild yourself and return to life. When you are in your mid 20's, it is never easy to come back to someone else's house and pick up where you left off, because you are not the same person anymore and neither is the place you left behind. But this is what reminds you that a good family is the backbone in your life and the eternal bonds of support that make you who you are. I have a feeling our girl is going to be just fine. She will find herself again, she will be stronger and wiser for all her experiences, and she will, ultimately, be able to move on and out into the world much better able to cope and manage all over again. For our part, our house will likely be a lot cleaner when she leaves again, our possessions nicely culled and her dad on his way back to good health. These are reasons to be cheerful. Her damaged heart will heal, and her spirits rise. She will come to understand that the road she was on was not the one the universe had planned for her. I told her not to be sad that it is over, but to be happy that it happened. That's what my fabulous Granny Myrtle told me on more than one occasion, having lost 3 husbands in her life, plus a crossroads where she nearly married the 4th, before he too keeled. Life is one long journey full of colorful pictures, events and people. Seldom do the same images and characters ride you through to the very end. "I thought we'd be together forever"; she cried to me. I reminded her that forever was a very long time and most of us don't get there.

(2020)

Friends are the family we choose

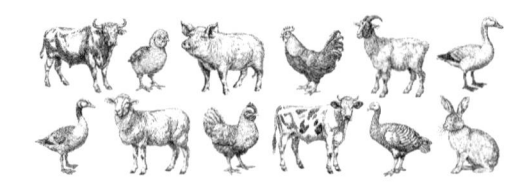

"Friends are the family we choose," she reminds me, as I am ranting on about some not unusual familial irritation in my daily life. "Oh, that must be why I enjoy being with my girls as much as I do," And I do, no word of a lie. Of course, I love my family a lot with all their warts and issues; but my friends are the total bomb. It's different with them; easy and fabulous. When we are apart, I crave for us to be together again. This past week I was so depressed because our incredible time together had yet again come to a close and I had to return home.

"Book the house for next May too!" I instruct our travel agent on the ground, who's always game for the next booking, the very next opportunity to laugh until she cries, the next date in the diary. And here we are almost a year out and I know she'll do it.

We have been constant friends since the age of 15 – truthfully, a very long time; and in some cases, a couple of divorces and a few kids ago. Some of us have lost siblings, others parents. We have cried through wretched diagnoses together and tough hands dealt. We have laughed uncontrollably for a good part of the last 40 years, so that is the very best thing of all. And we still make plans together all the time, dates in the diary for this year and next, though we live on different continents. We even do new and different things together when we meet up again – pony riding through the forest and river-tide-kayaking, thanks Kate, and seeking a San Fran exhibition that didn't exist in who-knows-where – thanks, Carey – and we now, increasingly, fantasize about the time in our lives when we are all widows, with our husbands dead and buried or cremated, and our children living out their lives and not wanting too much of our annoying selves around them. Not to say we are looking forward to any of those things; but let's be realistic here!

We have decided that we will all live together – likely in a nice house on the East Coast of England where I grew up, and where we are always planning our next reunion. It may be a dream, but it's a good one and not without possibility. We have all just returned from such a reunion in a multi-level home with private sea views and the most divine amount of sitting and enjoying spaces you could hope for in a single property. At one time, we were 7 or 8 in the house, easy-peasy, no drama … and I so didn't want to leave. I never want to leave.

"We'll likely need scooters by then," the conversation continues, when we are all home again and still talking about our golden years and our shared accommodations that we are already planning. "No one in their right mind will let us drive real vehicles by then!" Almost immediately, through the ether, came a selection of groovy scooter choices, each with its own personality just like us. Carey will need 1950's fins on hers, along with a matching outfit and sizable shopping basket or two. Kate will need some kind of rough-roading type of scooter – I'm thinking 3 wheels – in case she needs to digress over the beach or marshes, or chase naughty ponies, you never know! Lucy will likely need learner plates for the life of the bike and some kind of duo doggie seat option or sidecar for the border collies they will likely have as part of their large and extraordinary family by the sea. It's a wonderful dreamscape. We watch the prices of the properties in the town of our fantasies daily, we laugh a lot, and we dream even more. It's all good. It could happen. Not that we wish our husbands dead; but one must plan accordingly. You know.

"Dad! Dad!" I email my father with a 'May Day, May Day' urgent call to action. "I've always loved that house – it's the perfect situation. Buy it for me, please Dad? It's only seven hundred and fifty thousand pounds …" Didn't even get a response. Doesn't he know how important this is to my golden years? Now we've found a 7-bedroom number with pool and sea views. Oh my. Who can we persuade to buy it for us and let us make payments bit by bit? Such fun you cannot have with real money.

Now we are planning Kate's daughter's wedding and how fun is that? The honorary aunties have all invited themselves, as you do when you can claim you were almost on scene when the little munchkins were born all those years ago. We are talking outfits – as if ours really mattered – and gifts, that **will** matter, not to mention good, hard cash. It will be so absolutely fabulous for us to be present on such a happy day and I'm sure the tears will flow along with the champagne.

Our plans and our dreams, in juxtaposition, keep me buoyant when the day to day can seem, on occasion, quite tedious. I'm sure we are not alone in that dilemma. Holidays are the best part of the working person's life. Dreams are the stuff that take you to other planets, where things are done differently. And friends; friends, they are the family you choose to take with you through life. They are your safe port in a storm, the soothing voice at the end of the line, your holiday buddy and maybe, in some cases, they could be your roomie and scooter buddy towards the end of your life.

And who says it couldn't happen?

(2019)

Happy Birthday, dear Rita!

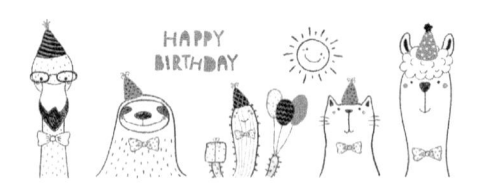

I hadn't seen her for a while, and when I did, I realized that she was very unwell. I was doing a book signing at a King City coffee shop and she was selling her amazing pies at the same venue. She had lost a lot of weight and had obviously started to struggle with her condition. I felt so badly for her. "Yeah, I've had this for about 25 years," she tells me with a wry smile. "Now they say it's time for a new liver!" I am no expert, but I could see that.

"I'll do it, Mum," my daughter tells me. "If it was my Mum needing a liver, I would hope someone would step up too." She was the right age and blood type. This could actually happen. I couldn't believe her generosity of spirit to put her own life on hold to help someone else's mother. And so, she put herself forward, completing all the necessary paperwork and counseling that was necessary. Her large heart scared me to pieces.

At the benefit for Rita's liver transplant in King City, I was so very delighted and amazed by how many people came out to support her and her family. The love in the room was tangible that night. Rita's very own famous pies raised $12,000 and $17,000 each in the Live Auction – yes for one pie, not a truckload! Literally tens of thousands of dollars were raised that evening to help the family get through this very difficult period in their lives – and, in addition; the living donor who might come along to save her life – our fingers and toes were firmly crossed for that miracle. The event also raised enormous awareness for the importance of being an organ donor, testing to be a liver donor in this case and how wonderful it is that the liver can regenerate itself so very quickly and completely. The parameters for being accepted as a donor were slim however, and most of her peers would not qualify. We were too old to be able to help, or with the wrong blood type. The clock was ticking swiftly on, and it was not in her favor.

It looked as if my daughter would be moving forward to the next stage of testing. She was required to spend a day up in Stanford and undergo a series of blood tests and then an MRI of the liver. I went along as her driver. I had never been to Stanford before. What a fascinating place – like a medical institution, but not really. An eerie calm pervaded the hallways, an air of distinguishment you don't experience in other medical buildings, but still it was entirely medical and, if you were in doubt of anything and looked around yourself, it was clear that we were surrounded by some very unwell looking folk – a bit of a dream sequence to be honest. As a potential donor, you don't pay anything for these tests, which is also very odd in the US. You hand over your health insurance card, but it won't be used. The check-in folk seemed surprised when my daughter presented herself as a potential donor, not that we know what an average donor looks like. I had read through all the info from Stanford about donating a liver and the science struck me as truly phenomenal. You can donate a portion of your liver to a person in need and you will be near back to normal within 2-3 months with that person's life saved. Their recovery will be even quicker than yours. Sounds simple, doesn't it.

It had been a very long day indeed once we stepped out of the campus at Stanford with the light fading. My daughter had donated 28 vials of blood and eaten nothing all day. That was likely the worst part of it for her.

It took a few days before they let her know that her liver levels were not healthy enough for her to be a donor and she was very disappointed. "I had wanted to do that for Rita," she expressed to me. Not to say she could not donate later, but for now she had to work on her own liver condition and get it back to a healthier state.

I immediately told Rita and she was so disappointed. All these roller coaster rides of getting hopes up and then for them to be quickly quashed and all the time she is feeling more and more unwell. There were a couple more donors tested and rejected before the message comes over on a Friday night. "She's been in surgery since 8am. 8–10-hour operation." What! What? Such joyous news and on her 60th birthday as well. A group of us who had been rallying around her – self-titled Team Rita – started bouncing off the walls. I couldn't eat my dinner. This was enormous news. We couldn't stand ourselves. "How is she?" "The operation went well", the message came back. "She is in recovery in ICU." Oh, that marvelous Stanford hospital, the selfless donor who must have had organ donor listed on their driving license or known to family and who was now saving Rita's life. So many thoughts scattered around my nighttime brain that I couldn't properly sleep or put my mind on a timeout. I wanted to deliver a large slice of virtual birthday cake to her and say, "See girl, just in time for your birthday, as we discussed!" Though the discussion had been around my girl's donation, not someone else's, the cheer is the same, the result equally fabulous. She is going to be okay.

Brooke, Josh, Paul and the rest of the family will be looking forward to celebrating many more birthdays and occasions with Rita. I cannot wait for the homecoming celebration when we can look her in the eye and already see the improved health coming back to her. It has been quite the journey for them all these past few years and now they will be able to look forward to some good health and happier days ahead.

If you have ever considered being an organ donor, please make it happen. What use will your organs be to you anyway, once your heart has stopped beating? I have my status as an organ donor firmly in place and my family knows my wishes. Please share this story of love and hope with anyone out there waiting for a miracle.

(2023)

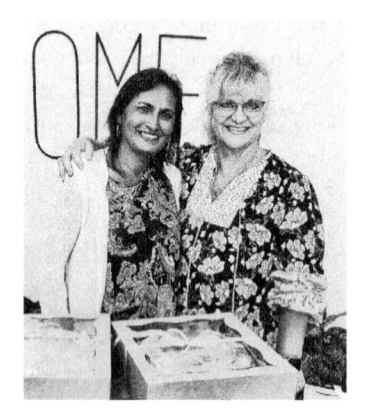

Rita & Lucy at the coffee shop

Her Anniversary

Even as I am feeling sad inside my head, louder I hear her voice ….. 'Oh for crying out loud, sister,' or words to that effect. "It's been blooming 4 years! Time to let me go and think about more interesting things." I wish I weren't such an anniversary hound, but that's not likely to change now. I remember driving my husband nearly potty when I used to remember the anniversary of our 1st date (still do), and he could barely even recall my birthday after 25 plus years together. He still has to very cautiously enquire *exactly* when our wedding anniversary is, as the day approaches. Some of us just have that memory gene, which can be a blessing as well as a curse.

As the 4th anniversary of Rosie's passing approached, I felt fractious and uptight. I felt angry and ripped off all over again, deeply sunken into a black mood. I dreamed about her and woke up missing her too much – all over again. So many self-righteous and entitled folk are still out here walking and breathing on our planet and my sister is now a mere skeleton wrapped in a blanket facing Allah on a Turkish hillside overlooking the bay of her home. True, her spirit swings around once in a while, like the host of dragonflies that flew before me in the road to lighten my load, or the divinest yellow butterfly near my head; but it's not enough, never enough. I couldn't put my finger on my renewed anger and freshly fertile grief except to say that, for some of us, a painful anniversary such as the passing of your baby sister, serves to rip the band-aid off the still tender wound and cause you to feel all those very difficult emotions all over again.

"4 years? I thought it was 3," said father. He's not one of the anniversary obsessives like me. Maybe no one is. I started work on my Rosie boat in the Secret Garden, my own personal memorial to her that I visit every day, but only touch up once a year. I couldn't find any wood glue to fix the letters of her name back on the boat. That made me cry. Yes, really. God, I was that fragile. Then I came home to 12 cream-colored roses from my husband who seldom buys flowers – and these were my wedding roses. I stopped in my tracks and realized that, though others can't tread the memory path the way I can, they are able to understand how difficult those days can be for me and that was so helpful that day. It almost assisted with the scab starting to heal over again. Friends of mine popped up and sent words of love, knowing that this transition through another anniversary was going to make everything raw and real again. My middle sister texted me that she knew I was going to have a tough day. She's not on the same memory go-around as me, but I know she struggles similarly through the difficult days – she just manages it better and would likely never cry over lost glue.

I couldn't finish a story that day, couldn't read a book or do anything useful. The wood glue was not found, so the Rosie boat was not repaired or repainted that day and I felt so guilty about that. How can you mark an important anniversary like that with a custom that you can't fulfil? Having not had the wood glue to hand, I had royally failed at that. What I did do was to take the day off and talk to her in my mind. I looked through photos, laughed at clips of old videos and was pretty self-indulgent the entire daylight hours. Me and her, her and me – it was our day. In the evening I drank a glass of good red and indulged in a bubble bath with a magazine. The next day it was back to regular life and work. I felt cleansed and better. I had survived another anniversary.

The wood glue was later purchased, and the Rosie boat restored to her former glory. Days later I had the courage to pick up my book about Rosie that I hadn't even looked at since it was published. I flicked through pages and laughed out loud at that girl. My goodness she was a hoot. So many lovely memories and great photos, moments in time encapsulated inside the 400 or so carefully written pages. And then some great grief lines in the back section that I'm quite proud of (Words of Sadness, Memory, Grief, Love and Solace) that bear repeating on occasion, since we all go through the stages of grief in our lives, not all memory hounds like me; but most of us, if we are honest, stumble through the process. Not well, I might add. My daughter's school friend was murdered last week in Nevada. My kid struggled immensely with this horrific news. "I hope she knew what a good friend she was to me," she tells me. "Tell her," I said. "Sit out under the stars and tell her." "I can't stop thinking about her," she said. "In my dreams, there were 5 coffins and I had to look in each one to find her." I hurt so deeply for her family left behind. Yes, grief, that thing, so difficult to navigate – no matter whether your loved one dies of a terminal illness or is murdered. Grief grabs you by the throat and throws you to the ground, pretty much without exception. Sometimes it holds you there for a very long time, sometimes you are thrown back into its mix by surprise – a song, a word, a memory, an anniversary. And there you are, back again, where you were before, drowning in waves of your own sorrow and gulping to come up for air. I also told my daughter to write a letter to her friend and then give it up to the universe. After Rosie died, I wrote several letters to her – a very therapeutic exercise. There are many tips inside my Rosie book for managing our grief and making appointments to meet with her at specific times.

'Well before Rosie passed away, I knew I would be writing her story – a patchwork quilt of her life. Little did I know what a therapeutic experience this would be for my own grieving process. When I got close to the end of the manuscript, I started to grieve just a little all over again.'

Me.

Grief never ends, but it changes. It's a passage, not a place to stay. Grief is not a sign of weakness, nor a lack of faith. It is the price of love.

(Author unknown)

Life happens ....

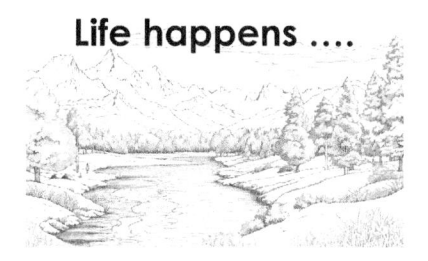

That was my Facebook post of a truck that was smashed beyond belief. It belonged to my daughter's boyfriend, Aaron, and my daughter was the passenger.

Saturday night and I was nicely snuggled with my granddaughter Madison. We were reading Junie B Jones together in bed. She's going to be a 1st grader, so this was the very wonderful *Junie B Jones, First grader: Cheater Pants* edition. We were roaring with laughter at that crazy girl. Special times.

I noticed a missed call from Aaron which struck a bit of an uneasy chord. They had left only a few hours ago for their 10-day, dream vacation in Montana. I call him back and those are terrifying sounds a mother cannot unhear. The screams of your child with the buzz of First Responders all around her in the background. They had been in a most horrific crash, and she was trapped in the wreckage. Everything froze. I paced the house. Up and down. Down and up. I could barely breathe. A wrong-way driver had hit them head-on on the freeway near Reading.

The hours after that are all a blur. The hours until I could actually see and hear her and note the wiggle of her toes and fingers. Truthfully, I'm not quite sure how I got to Vacaville. They were still doing MRI's and X-rays when I got there; but it was clear she had broken her back.

I had heard about Kaiser hospitals before and how special they were. In Kaiser Vacaville, Francoise had her own room without the usual hospital noises and chaos that you expect under normal hospitalization situations. They let her boyfriend and I stay in the room with her (he wasn't physically injured) and treated us like family. They knew we weren't patients, but we were hurting all the same. They offered us coffee and kindness. From the CNA Rachel, (can we adopt you?) to the nutritionist Jessica (oh how cute and kind you were to us, we didn't want to leave you!) to the tip-top RN Glenn who was so particular and thoughtful in his treatment of my daughter that you would have thought she was his only patient, and to the head nurse Maria (a mango a day will be in my mantra forever ..) and many others. I have never been sad to leave a hospital before; but this time I really was. We felt so safe there; that her recovery was in their capable hands and their hands were so good.

Come to find out, an old friend of mine from Soledad was now working up at that hospital. She came to visit us and gave us good advice about what we should do. Being in the medical world, she was a big help and steered us in the right direction. We needed that, as adrift as we were at the time. The next day she returned with cupcakes baked by her daughter. So very cheering! Thank you, Stephanie and Alyssa! Familiar faces in the storm are such a comfort. Another old friend lives close by and she visited us with yummy coffees after work. Cheers to Thais, the lovely Wonder Woman! Our son Marc came from Sacramento bearing the most delicious tamales in the world and took Aaron under his wing to deal with the destroyed vehicle and police report. Aaron could not have managed that alone; it's so distressing to revisit the scene of the crime, as it were, and so nice to be reminded of the basic kindness and humanity of people when you really need them. So many folks in Facebook land asked what they could do to help. We felt so wrapped in love and support.

She's home now. She was so traumatized by the accident it took me a while, days even, to be able to get her into the car. Every time we tried it, her blood pressure would crash, she'd feel nauseous, and her pain would soar. Then Glenn would smile, tell us she wasn't ready yet and put her back to bed. Finally, we managed our escape with an accompaniment of pillows and drugs. Rockstar Nurse Glenn wheeled her out from the cocoon of the hospital, room 307, to the big world outside. Truthfully, we wanted to take that guy home with us; but he had other lives to save, other families to cheer along – not to mention his own family of a wife and 5 kids.

My daughter's rollercoaster road to recovery is meshed with a good deal of anger and sadness. Their beautiful and special vacation was destroyed by a drugged or negligent driver; we don't know which yet. Aaron's truck is obliterated, along with many of their prized possessions. Her back is broken, everything fun has had to be canceled. She is likely not able to start her nursing school on time or go to any of the concerts they had planned in the coming days and weeks. Her fury towards the mystery perpetrators currently knows no bounds. We remind her of how lucky she is to be alive and not paralyzed; but that is little comfort to her during these early days of grief and fury; not to mention pain.

One thing she does know, for sure, is that Aaron has been by her side every minute of every day since the accident. When it happened, he jumped out of the truck, called 911, and rushed to hold her head steady, also her heart, while the first responders cut her out of the vehicle. The days after he didn't leave her side, not even once. The hospital crew joked that he needed to put on a pair of scrubs and help them out in his spare time. He did everything for my girl from bathing her to massaging her feet and cheering her spirits. He didn't sleep for days in case she needed him. As I commented to one of my friends, "true love can be found in the shattered glass of broken dreams."

In the meantime, the flowers, friends and meals keep arriving at our house, (thank you Jessica, Anthony, Precila and Fabian!) It all helps. Our girl is practicing her walking, getting stronger every day, and the VNA will be coming next week to check her out and move along her physical therapy. Two kittens will be arriving to cheerlead her recovery – nothing like a kitten to lift the spirits – and we, her family, will be at her side for whatever she needs in the coming days, as she rebuilds her body and spirits. "This is a life-altering experience," she tells me. Yes. Sometimes life gives us those too.

"One of our greatest freedoms is how we react to things," said the mole to the boy.

'What do we do when our heart hurts?" asked the boy.

"We wrap them with friendship, shared tears and time, till they wake hopeful and happy again," said the horse.

"Nothing beats kindness," said the horse. "It sits quietly beyond all things."

"Sometimes," said the horse.

"Sometimes what?" asked the boy.

"Sometimes just getting up and carrying on is brave and magnificent."

The Boy, the Mole, the Fox and the Horse
By Charlie Mackesy

Thanks to all who helped us, loved us, and made sure we didn't fall to the ground this week, never to rise again. We are not yet put back together; nor are we broken. Marginally fractured might be a better description. We so appreciate all the love.

(2021)

Love is all that matters

I've never got hung up on Fathers, Mothers, Sisters, Brothers … if we grew up together, then you are mine, and sometimes you are mine if we didn't. Most of my family are bits and pieces from all over the place and I think that makes for a most interesting melting pot, a pond full of diversity – indeed the makings of a very fabulous life.

My father adopted me when I was about 4 years old. In those days, the adoptions were closed, and everything was much more uptight than it is today. When I was a rebellious teenager and my mother refused to share any info with me, I traced my natural father and his family who, oddly enough, lived up the road from us in the sizeable City of London. He was a pastor. I never met him, but he was reportedly quite a character. When I came to later know Dominic, one of his son's, he told me that I was fortunate I didn't grow up in their family. His dad was so busy saving the world, he forgot to take care of his own children. The nicest thing he ever said to Dominic was that he was the best traveled member of his family.

And fortunate is exactly how I feel. I was always treated the same as my sisters and we had a wonderful childhood. Our father worked long hours to keep everything just so for us and our mother was able to stay at home and do important things like reading and art with us that became important foundations for our future lives. She was a talented artist and, though she was a harsh critic of her own work, fostered a wonder for the artistic world in us that appeared in various ways. My sister Rosie was a superb artist herself, Mary a highly well-read academic and me … well a bit of writing here, a bit of photography there, a little music … all pursuits completely endorsed by our parents. We attended private schools and received the best education, though I wish I had done something a little more career-driven with mine. Our middle sister Mary recently completed her training as an attorney at the ripe old age of 50 plus and is dutifully employed with a law office. It's all good. We arrive in our happy places at different stages in life. Our father retired from 30 plus years with his father's company and then went back to school, where he flourished in his academia and made life-long friends.

My 2nd husband adopted my daughter when she was about 5 years old. Things were now much more free and easy in the world in that regard and we were able to have fun with the adoption. As a blended family of two older boys and one younger girl, it was an insane mish-mash that consisted of the most delicious chaos. We had an adoption party for our daughter, and she got to wear a Princess dress and tiara. My husband gave her a ring and his family gave her a necklace. We had the most delightful adoption party in the park with all the relatives in attendance. My daughter has never been hung up about adoption either. When her natural father attempted contact a few years later, she told me she had no interest in him or his family. I showed her a photo or two and she was satisfied. It seemed like a healthy response to me, though I didn't force the issue either way. Not my choice to make. She knows what she has with her only dad, and it goes way beyond any blood lines. They are the best of friends and deeply loving towards one another.

My husband's sons went back and forth between their mother and father in the early days of their divorce, and it was a most difficult period for them. I inherited them at the tricky ages of 11 and 13, so that made for some interesting times. Their mother was not a very balanced person and created lots of turmoil for those formative minds in the early days. I could not be their mother – they had one of those – but I could be their friend and adviser, a role I took on with little knowledge of the male species. Gradually I came to realize that they would call or consult me before their father, and I took on my own position of importance in their lives. When their mother died, I didn't try and push anything, but attempted to be comforting and consoling and continue my job as their friend and supporter. We treat all our children the same, just as my parents did. Both my sisters have had similar supporting roles with their husbands' children, and I see a familiarity among us of being the safe harbor in the storm for the children, the comfy sofa when all around feels a bit rocky. I think we have served our positions as stepmothers admirably, unattractive title that it is. And now I have a granddaughter and she claims me and me her. It doesn't matter ultimately where all these souls came from. Love is all that matters.

This Father's Day, my daughter took her dad out fishing to a nearby lake. There's a lovely photo of the two of them sitting on their fishing stools and chatting away, as they are wont to do. They are so comfortable in each other's space. My son is also taking his daughter out fishing for the day. I'm proud to say that he is a good dad as well.

If you are in a blended family that struggles to mesh the way you should, put yourselves in the shoes of the other person and try to be as mellow and accepting as possible. It will likely serve you well. Though I never anticipated that I would raise two boys from teenage-dom (and continue *raising* them per se in adulthood, because we are never done, are we!) I would have laughed out loud. We didn't have boys in our family. As dad fondly joked – even our family dog was a female. There was no escaping the estrogen levels in our house.

I love all my children, as they do me – I believe. And, again, love is all that matters.

Thanks to my dad for all you have done and continue to do for me and my family. You are much loved.

(2020)

Motherhood is not for wimps.

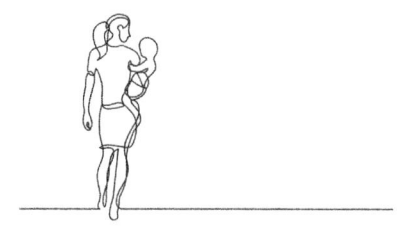

How is my child now more than a quarter century old? It sometimes feels as if it was yesterday that she popped into the world. I recall so clearly the labor – 24 hours and counting in all, before they cut her out of me, (when initially I thought I had indigestion, the bane of my pregnancy!) I recall my father driving me to the hospital in the back of my red Nissan. I think he was going about 5 miles an hour with this 200lb beast – me – cussing and writhing in the back seat. I also recall my mother trying to make me eat before we left for the labor ward – ever the European Mama, insisting that a good meal would solve everything. I seem to remember it was beef stew she was trying to feed this poor monster in labor.

And then once I saw her, the world stood still. No matter they had cut through 18 layers of skin to get at her, and my body systems were all messed up when her blood got into mine due to our different blood types. None of that mattered when I saw her and discovered that she was *normal*. I had made it through and so had she. Then the healing could begin.

Before I had my daughter, I had never once changed a diaper; not something I'm particularly proud of, but it's the truth. I had not been what you might call a maternal type. I didn't babysit infants or covet the idea of being a Mum as my life goal. Friends of mine had mothered already and suggested that you have to have at least one; but I was left unmoved by all their persuasions. I was quite happy with my dogs, thank you very much. But when she showed up, the only thing I felt was the complete and utter pureness of love. I saw her perfect face; her dark hair and blue eyes and I was instantly smothered with adoration. She was mine and I was hers and that was all there was to it. I remember my Mum telling me something similar.

Having had no practice at any of the early day stuff, I relied entirely on friends who had done it before. Thank goodness, there were some super handy types close by who had graduated that particular class and were able to coax me along. As a new and clueless mother, I was stumbling through the dark.

The early years were tiring but fabulous. She was so hilarious and curious about the world. She had funny habits … who eats one cheerio at a time? Who will go to a restaurant and want only ice? Who will not be able to walk on sand or grass? Yes, that would be my girl. Fortunately, when she turned about 1.5 years, I met my life partner and this was not his first parenting rodeo, so he started guiding me towards the light and helping me to navigate those early years when 'no!' is the favored word of a toddler, closely followed by '*I don't want to!*'

The later years might be diagnosed as a little bit of a challenge; but most of us old mothers agree that it wouldn't be normal otherwise. You can't just have bliss-bliss all the way through. They would never leave home and you would never want them to. She went through all the teenage tussles that most of us do – (though she wasn't a patch on her naughty Auntie Rosie!) She came through to the other side and then we would do fun things together, instead of fighting. We would travel, go to concerts and have fun wherever we went. We still do. We will plan a fun day out – lunch, shopping, sometimes a mani-pedi. We haven't traveled together for a while, since, yeah, no one has been able to do much of that; but everything we do together is so memorable. I realized, thinking about her birthday, that she and I are mostly the best of friends. Sometimes I get on her nerves, ('Are you home for dinner? Did you have fun? Did you eat? …' you know, annoying mother banter.) Sometimes she gets on my nerves and me on her last nerve; but as I have reminded her time after time; she is mine and I am hers, and there is no amount of annoyingness that is going to change that. I promised not to be a burden on her in my later years … who needs that kind of garbage in their lives. And I promised to try to not ask too many annoying questions while we are, likely temporarily, sharing the same roof. But one thing we do know for sure is that I will love her forever, regardless, and she me. My own mother has been gone from this planet over 2 decades and I will still love her forever. It's the rite of passage, the way to be and the absolute blessing of a mother-daughter relationship. We fight like sisters on occasion; we will spit at each other like llamas; but the love is deeply entrenched. We are part of the same tree, a branch each of the other. I am hers and she is mine.

My friends were right way back when, a hundred years ago – or at least a couple decades – when they told me you do need to have at least one – not necessarily birthed the uncomfortable way I did it, because there are many ways to bring a child into your life, without all the 24-hour labor pains some of us endured. My daughter has driven me crazy in a whole host of ways over the years and I have been crazy in love with her since I first saw her; so that's not likely to change much, as she evolves into a beautiful adult in her own right and I'm happy to watch her go there.

It's stunning to watch her develop as a mature and kind person. My friend describes her as an old soul, and she is that. I see my grandmother in her and my baby sister too. The middle sister is there also and, once in a while, she has the tongue of my mother and the innate kindness of my father. I see all kinds of strands within her, and it is a delight to behold.

Thank you, Universe, for letting me be her mother. It's been quite the job, but not one I would have missed for the world.

Francoise Kallista Liberty Mason Jensen is my baby girl, and she just celebrated another birthday.

(September 2020)

Sister Sheryl

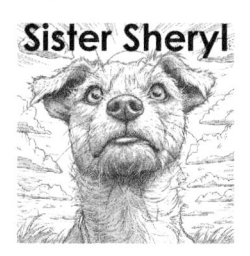

Our first meeting was an interesting one. I had been hired as her boss at the local paper. She took me to see one of her oldest friends and clients. I was told by the customer, in no uncertain terms, that if I took her away as this client's advertising lady, she would no longer advertise. That's the kind of loyalty she inspired in this and many, many other customers of the newspaper. Of course, I wasn't going to change out her rep! Who would make that kind of mistake on their first day at the office!

It was so nice when the paper group still used the Soledad Bee office next to mine. We could just catch up over a cup of tea, or I could go in there and pillage old stories of mine I had misplaced or get the scoop on local happenings. But times change, as they do, and the Bee office closed.

I was only her boss per se for about 5 minutes and then I changed my job from newspaper to real estate, but we remained firm friends. Over the years, we would visit each other in hospital – there's friendship for you – we would show up to each other's stuff (thank you for always coming to my book signings and making this local author feel as if people really do still read books!) We would enjoy a lunch occasionally at the little hometown Mexican restaurant equidistant from our two offices, where we would catch up on the prior months and do a little late birthday or Christmas celebration. We would always just jump right in there where we left off. How are the kids and the grandkids? How's the paper world? Yes, of course I have another book coming out. You know – old friend banter.

She adopted a little black scrawny dog from SCAR when the charity was first starting out. Originally, she was just going to foster the pooch, but her big old heart would have bust at the seams if she'd had to say goodbye, so she took her in full time. "I can't foster," she told me. "I'd have to keep them all!" But she was always an enormous supporter of the rescue anyway and helped out when she could. I loved seeing her at the SCAR and Soledad Museum tea party fundraisers. She would come with her grandchildren, and I think they loved it nearly as much as she did! In fact, she was an enormous supporter of all kinds of needy causes, quietly helping with ad costs or buying tickets or working behind the scenes. I got to sit with her and her bestie at the Rita Tavernetti fundraiser in the spring and it was so fun to sit and break bread with her of an evening (also the most luscious tiramisu known to man that she purchased for the table at the cake walk.)

Sister Sheryl as her old friend and advertiser always calls her is retiring from the newspaper business in the coming days. I couldn't believe it when she told me the news. I thought she would always be there, like an institution that could never close its doors. But change comes to all and even newsies get to retire on occasion. I am super happy for her – she so deserves some peace and quiet and beach time that she loves and doesn't get enough of – but I'm sad for all of us. For 22 years, she has loyally and diligently serviced clients and friends with her happy voice and big hugs. She has been a constant in the local newspaper world that has known little constancy these past few years. She reminds me of my deadlines and reminds me again when I am still forgetting my deadlines. She listens to me when I need to vent, she helps me when I'm down. Yeah, one of those kinds of friends. And I'm sure many people feel that way about her.

Fortunately, she won't be leaving the area, so we will still be able to meet for cups of tea or Mexican food and kick the dust, share the scoop. I imagine she will have more time to cruise with the besties now and love on her beautiful grandchildren. I told her that the title of my next book of columns is going to be *Tomorrow is not promised*, and she liked that. She gets the concept. She will soon be enjoying her today and her tomorrows without the pressures of work and deadlines.

Thank you, Sheryl, for all the years and the friendship. I know you are leaving your considerable desk in good hands, and I do hope you will still remind me of my deadlines, check my ads and read my stories.

Much love –

Your advertiser and friend,

Lucy

XX

Sisters

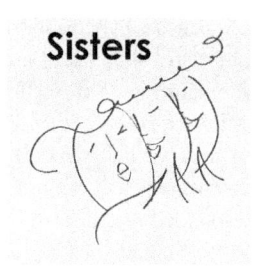

We were always the slices of bread separated by her jam filling. She was the youngest, the naughtiest, the most demanding of the family's attention. There wasn't much more than a year between the youngest and the middle, so it always felt as if there were the 3 of us, with the youngest being the most high-maintenance child. That was the dynamic we grew up with and became accustomed to. The baby sister's various surgeries to fix her congenital hip as a youngster was just the prelude to all that would come in adulthood. From age 32 on, until her death at 48, it was all about Rosie. We would travel from wherever the rest of us lived on the planet to where Rosie's home was in Turkey, as you do when a family member has a nasty disease, and they really cannot travel.

Dad's birthday would be celebrated with all of us together in Turkey. It was always the last summer, the last birthday, as the middle sister noted a little wryly while baby sister was alive – *The Longest Goodbye* – as it can be when you are continuing to live with Stage 4 cancer and enjoying the benefits of life extensions through developments in medical research. As the youngest proudly observed, on more than one occasion, 'I am a miracle of science!' And then there was nothing more they could do for her; her liver was shot, and the miracle began to fade. I could feel that the family dynamic was about to dramatically alter. I warned our dad that our family unit was about to become fractured; that we had lived 48 years with that demanding, sparky little spitfire and how were we going to manage without her?

A few days after she died, I wrote to my middle sister that I would try and be a better sister from now on. For so long it had always been about the youngest, I wondered what we would find to talk about, whether the years of not paying much attention to each other would have permanently damaged our sisterhood. We had not visited each other's homes in years, we didn't know much about the other's lives. Without anything conscious, we had somehow managed to bypass one another because of our commitment to our ill sister. She was the filling to our bread. And then our plates shifted.

They say that about a terrible illness in the family; that it can absorb the other family members, so they become almost unimportant in the larger scheme of things. In their efforts to save and support the life of the one sibling in need, they are nearly invisible. And it's true; it happens by default. And then the high maintenance child is gone and the other two start emerging cautiously from the shadows. Grief can be a great separator; I've found in the past. But this time it was different. I admitted to middle sister that I had crashed pretty badly after baby sister's death, and this was the beginning of us finding our way back to each other. Though our reactions were different, our feelings of loss were similar. We had to learn to continue on with our lives, always remembering that sparky little pistol, but still living our lives and carrying on and doing our best to be happy.

And then Middle Sister decided to come and stay for a week at my house – she hadn't visited in several years. We had such a lovely time together, discounting the clumsy falls each one of us had – me in Monterey and her in the vineyard! We stayed in nice hotels, ate delicious food, swam and played with the puppies. It was a super special time, and we didn't want it to end. The next plan is that I am taking our father over to her home for Christmas and I haven't been there since her wedding several years ago; I haven't been in England over the holiday season for ions either. So, lots of positive things have come out of our youngest sister's death, as she would certainly have hoped and anticipated. This week we celebrate our birthdays – exactly 5 years apart – and I'm so glad that we have been able to reconnect. Families are certainly a work in progress, as are most relationships; but I have a feeling that ours is going to be just fine. Though we will always miss our naughty little sister and things in our world are certainly quieter without her, it is good to share the memories and the photos and keep her alive in that way.

(2019)

So much love

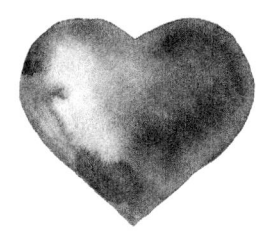

Anybody want a humongous house for 12 people, 3 nights in Bozeman Montana? A 49er game with parking for 4 (oh, yes please .. wait. I was outbid). How about a 7 day stay in Copper Mountain, Colorado? A 48-hour wild pig hunt, maybe, or a steak dinner with all the trims and drinks for 8 at Grace's place? You do? Sorry, you're too late. You should have been the top bidder at the live auction of the Rita Tavernetti liver transplant benefit, where the people came out for one of their own and bought their money with them. Boy, did they. King City is world-famous for that. From coveted peanut brittle to pies (Rita's very own apple pies commanded a casual $17,000 and $12,000 each – 2 pies only, not a truck load – during the live auction!) It was a beautiful sight to behold. People helping people, such a concept; but pretty much par for the course in the City of King.

From its inception a few short months ago, the fundraiser for Rita and her as-yet undesignated liver donor, seemed as if it was going to be a popular event. You don't grow up in an area and be vested in schools, business and community without picking up a few friends and fans along the way; but I have honestly NEVER seen so many decorated tables for a banquet as we did that night in the Orradre building. Every little detail was accounted for and checked off the list by the many dedicated volunteers for the benefit. The steak dinner was delish (Thank you, King City Young Farmers), the auction – live and silent – outstanding, (also so overwhelming I forgot one of the items I won. The Auction's crew outdid themselves) – the bar swift and fabulous – and the company, oh so good. Even my husband enjoyed himself and he'd always rather be at home with the animals than out in the community.

Love was the theme of the night and so many people mentioned that. Rita herself said "it was an incredible evening – so many people and so much love." Matt Gourley nailed it pretty spot-on with his comment, "What an amazing community effort! The love in the room was astounding." Yes, it was Matt, and I think we all felt the magic in the room that evening. Nights like that make you honored to be a part of a community that can inspire such empathy and compassion for a fellow human.

So, yes, indeed, thank you for an incredible job well done by all and buckets of money raised, (the bean counters are still counting). And now for the somber tone that needs to be repeated. Rita does not yet have an accepted liver donor. Many have thus far tested, so it is not for want of trying. It is obviously a very slim window of people that can be considered for further testing beyond the basic parameters. For starters, you must be O- or O+ blood type, under 55 years old (darn) and in good health. Many of us have 2 out of the three qualifications required, but there is no requirement waiver available for this. The liver is an amazing organ that regenerates – I have learned so much about it through Rita's journey. The donor's liver will fully recover very quickly after donation – did you know that? The procedure is not massively invasive – who knew? You are saving someone's life – beyond words. And so, the real work starts now to try and get more people to test, more people to call up Lourdes at Stanford and say 'Hey, I just think I might be a match for Rita!' (Lourdes is the transplant coordinator at Stanford. Let's hope she gets inundated with people within the correct framework who want to test!)

And, then we wait, and the waiting is the hardest. I have known Rita for many years, our paths have crossed at all kinds of intersections in life and we are, best of all, friends. Good friends, old friends. But now she needs more than friendship – she needs my help, your help, everyone's help. And, in this rather pushy, bossy, insistent way, I feel sure, together, we can find her donor angel. As a village – the one I saw at the benefit – we can all find the lifesaver that will bring Rita back to her full life in the community she loves so well with her beloved family and friends at her side.

I'm hoping that you can share this tale of generosity, hope and love with others in your circle. As my daughter so succinctly put it, "if it was my Mum needing a liver, I hope people would come out and test for her!" And, yes, my daughter is testing. At least, she has the age part right, which many of us don't, and the blood type too. Maybe she will become Rita's angel and make this quest one of ultimate success all the way around. And I don't say this to brag on my daughter, a local nurse no less; but I say it to encourage you to push your loved ones forward as well. If I can contemplate and accept my daughter doing this for Rita, then perhaps you can do the same. I trust in the science, and I trust in the skills of the doctors at Stanford. I also trust in the power of love to lift up all who need it and make tough situations right, the sick well and the struggling resolved.

There have been a lot of tears shed recently and a lot of hugs and love shared in this close room that is our community. Now we need to find THE donor for Rita so she can get the surgery she so desperately needs.

Together, I know we can make this happen for Rita and her family. Boots on the ground, troops on alert. It's time for Rita to get the surgery. A donor must be found.

Thanks for reading and sharing and pulling up a chair to my table.

Love,

Lucy

(PS In June 2023 an angel donor was found, and, to date, Rita is doing so very well.)

The Dump Trailer

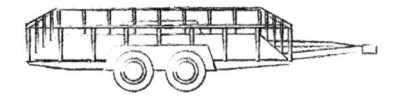

You know you are middle-aged, or frankly on the wrong side of the bridge, if you get excited about a dump truck. We'll just call him Scotty. Right at the beginning of our remodel of sorts, we looked around at our precious piles of *assets* oozing out of the orifices at our home called Solace and literally gasped. Over 20 years we had accumulated so much stuff, our little house was over-brimming with these *assets* (I use the term lightly!) And then, if you add land to the equation, you can find yourself in a right pickle. Land equals more places to put stuff. No one blinked when we added another *storage* building to the back 40, or did an extension on the garden shed, or man-cave as it came to be known (note to self, if you put a recliner in the man-cave, the cats will use it for all kinds of things.) We were literally falling over *essential items* that we might, possibly, find a use for one day. My daughter would point at the screen of the show *Hoarders* when it came on and tell us, like an intervention of sorts, "this is you two."

In our defense, we were both raised in thrifty households, where nothing was ever thrown away. I've always considered myself *messy* at best – my mother's fault entirely – because she was super messy. Prior to buying our house up in the Gabilans about 20 years ago, we were renters and had moved consistently over the years, so we never had time to gather possessions. It was time. No excuses. Scotty had become a necessity in our lives.

Husband took some time looking for the perfect Scotty and, come to find out, the pandemic meant that Scotties had become very expensive and were hard to find. Who knew! Everyone had decided they were hoarders and were clearing out their assets! Either that or a trip to the dump was like a legal outing when everyone was on lockdown. Laughable really. Once we started looking for dump trailers, we saw them everywhere, literally everywhere. "Ooooh look", he'd gasp, "that's a beauty with an auto dump feature as well!" An auto dump feature? Gawd, we had become ancient old fogies. No longer excited about the classic Camaro or the swish and sexy new leather jacket … no, we were on the lookout for the perfect dump trailer. And there he was. We scooped him up like eager adoptive parents and took him home, where he had to receive, primarily, a lock feature so that no one would steal him. Oh, it's a thing apparently.

And poor old Scotty has received such a workout these past few weeks, we have no idea how we managed without him. Our son and daughter in law in Switzerland love to go to the dump when they visit. They enjoy all the gulls and chaos of the dirt-moving machines, the auto dump feature, (delightful, they laugh every time), oh and the sheer joy of driving a load of trash around the streets. Who knew, Scotty would become such a popular member of the family!

And to those of you who think you don't need a Scotty in your lives; you're wrong. Either you own a Scotty, or you borrow a Scotty. It's as simple as that.

(2020)

The Mehs

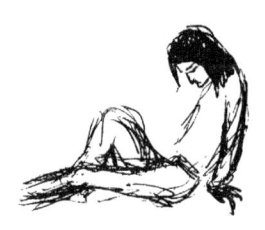

Well, I had a case of the 'mehs' … something you see a lot on social media these days, if you cruise around the world of Instagram, Snap Chat et al. in this modern world of communication. I have asked my daughter, on occasion, how she is doing and sometimes, I just get a *meh* in response over text. It's a new word. I'm sure my parents would not have allowed it in one of our hard-fought Scrabble games of yore, but, as of 2019, it's a word. Google tells me it's an exclamation that expresses a lack of interest or enthusiasm. So that's what I had; all of that. I could barely put one foot in front of the other – that's how *meh-y* I felt. The sun was shining, the dogs were playing, the llama was strutting around on the deck, I was not ill. Why did I feel this way? I do my best to stay very busy these days. When I am not working in the office, for the animal rescue, or working at home, I have plans to be working on something. I rarely stop. On the weekends, I seem to push myself harder than even during the week. It's an absolute necessity that I am completely worn out at night, so I do not just go to sleep; I cascade into slumber, my body exhausted. It's called getting through the first year, apparently.

I communicated with one of my oldest friends in England. "I've got the mehs," I told her. "Yeah, me too." She responded. "I've been flat on my back with a bad back, on pain meds and not much else. I'm so sick of myself. "All of a sudden, I realized that my back was working perfectly fine thank you very much and I should not be attending my own private pity party, when important people in my life were suffering. I was physically fine, just a bit *meh-y*. "Get over yourself," I told myself and started working on another project to keep the dark thoughts at bay and myself keeping on, as they say.

I decided to buy my friend some goodies and package them up, as good friends do. There's nothing quite like an honest-to-goodness mystery parcel in the post to give you a lift. I would include all her favorite American sweeties and a couple of books, a few uplifting or funny. She will be so happy, I anticipate. Her back will, suddenly, feel totally restored. Off I went, proudly, with my goodies all parceled up and my customs form completed. 'What a nice friend,' I told myself, as I trucked on over to the post office. "That will be $67.80," he tells me. "Or $85.60 priority." What? She'd be furious if I sent her a parcel of cheer that cost so much to ship, so I told her instead I was sending her a *virtual gift* … she wouldn't actually be receiving it in the post, but the intention had been there, and she would get it the next time our paths crossed. It's even still wrapped! Oh, we had a giggle about that. A virtual gift! What next? Mehs and a virtual gift. My mother would think she was living on a different planet!

It's been a year since I was last in Turkey with my sister, our last days together on the planet. Next month will be a year since her passing. It's not an easy time for my family. "Get through the first year," they say. "It's better after that." I'm not so sure about better, but I do know that time eases things and the memories become eventually sweeter and less painful. We all miss her keenly in different ways. My father and I were talking about it being tennis season and how they used to love to talk about the tennis matches they had watched and what was coming up. I know he has been feeling a large, quiet gap there. We also talked about her years of treatment, how she had been in England for her chemo, January of 2004, and how she did pottery while she was there. Randomly, the same day, an old email pops up from her to me, as I'm digging through a box of letters.

January 28, 2004,

Dearest Lucia,

Well, the day has come when hair is falling out in big clumps and I'm going to get my head shaved. I think it is socially unacceptable to trail and drop hair everywhere. It comes from everywhere, so waxing is a thing of the past. It has some advantages then this chemo thing. Well have been continuing the ceramic painting and today finished a beautiful fish plate ...

Have meeting at Cancerkin young woman's group tomorrow afternoon, which will be interesting, looking forward to sharing head care facts with people, like should one moisturize bald pate?...

I could hear her perky cheery voice, still full of laughter – regardless – and my heart was instantly so full of love that I forgot to be sad. Strange also that I am working on my next project about my amazing baby sis, her cancer, our sisterhood of cancer and more. Maybe some more jewels from the past will fall in my lap on my journey to, eventually, creating something special in her memory.

Like a brief storm that passes through, the 'mehs' are gone and I'm back to working on something constructive again.

Thanks for the kick in the tush, Bud. I could always count on you to cheer me up – or, at least, to get over myself for a little while.

(2019)

The move to Montana

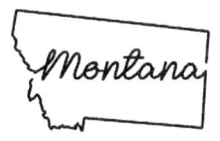

"We'll be moving to Montana," she said matter of fact. "How exciting, darling!" I expressed and, yes, it would be exciting for them. For me too, as I would have a new place to visit. I recall so clearly, when I moved to the Central Coast, that my folks were delighted. They would have a new part of the world to explore; and they certainly took full advantage of that. Wherever I was living at the time – and it mostly certainly was never Carmel Village – that is where they would stay, even down to the same Inn and sometimes room. They would eat at the same places and enjoy the same walks. Though they were really coming to visit me, they made the very best of their time and adored their holidays here on this beautiful coast. At the end of her life, my mother told me that if she could go back to one more place in the world, it would be to Monterey. (Another reason I transported her ashes – First Class, no less – back to the Monterey Bay.) Even now that my dad can't travel, he loves to hear about the places we go on the Central Coast, being able to pinpoint them on a map and in his memory. Eventually his ashes will join my mother's and some of mine will join them in due course.

I digress. Apparently, my daughter and her boyfriend will be moving to Montana where he's from. Just not this week. Ever since they rented their home, which they call the Hacienda, they have been gathering family members like there's no tomorrow. As of today, they have 2 dogs, 2 cats, 2 pigs and, I think, 6 goats. "How are you going to transport all your menagerie to Montana?" I ask of her with some validation. "Oh, you know, a trailer or two, dad …" her voice drifts off. As it stands right now, whenever she needs a dog sitter for her enormous Great Pyrenees pony Moose, she calls on her dad. When she needs to pick up pallets or whatever she needs really, she calls on her dad. I joked with the husband that he will need to figure out the best way to get to Montana in the quickest possible time, because our daughter is not known for her patience and need him she will, wherever she ends up laying her head!

"How are you going to manage in Montana without your dad being at your beck and call?" I ask cautiously. "Oh, you guys will be coming too!" Ha, I nearly choked on my coffee at that point. I like to visit different spots on the planet; it doesn't mean I'd want to live there! I think I would adore Montana in the spring and fall. The summers and winters don't look like they are quite up my alley and especially not the long, white winters. A little dusting on the Santa Lucias is quite enough snow for me. But you raise your children so that they can successfully live without you and maybe raise their own; so, I would never honestly challenge her wish to move to Montana. We must all experience the world for ourselves just like I did. My parents never once questioned my move to America or how much I might need them when I got there.

On the latest adventure to the pallet shed with the truck and trailer, she announces that they are going to be building chicken pens. Ah, the menagerie is growing! I chuckle at her ever-increasing farm (the apple doesn't fall too far from the tree) and her equally similar lust for adventure. "Another tow trailer to add to the 3 you will already need for the trip, plus dad?" I jest.

"You do know that Montana has really long, cold winters, right?" I enquire. "Oh, I know. We may just make some trips there instead," she responded, smiling.

"Well, if you want a large ranch, that would be the place," I put another possible dreamscape into her brain, and she just smiled. Nice to be young and free and able to ponder the next move, maybe, perhaps, just around the corner, perhaps later, perhaps never.

In the meantime, she lives only 30 minutes away from Solace and she and her boyfriend love their Hacienda with all their critters. They have good jobs, lovely plans and a nice life. Your quest in life is for your children to be happy and I do believe she is. That makes Mama Bear very happy in her turn and optimistic that the future will be fine, whether it happens here or there or somewhere in between. Moving to Montana? May happen, may never. That's one of the joys of life. The best-made plans seldom go in the originally planned direction.

(2023)

The navigation of grief

It has been 2 years since my baby sister Rosie passed on to another planet. When some say that spirits fly close to the ground, I have found that to be true – also that they don't fly in the conventional sense. Sister seems to pass through my aura not at my bidding but when she darn well feels like it; typical of her. I watch her flutter by as a white butterfly, I attach myself to the wings of summer dragonflies and talk to them as I would talk to her, I find her often times in the water; I try and drag her back to our planet in whatever form I can recognize.

Milestones of grief are difficult to navigate; especially when the loss is fresh. To get through the often-agonizing days, you hold tight to your friends and family who know how you are feeling, really know. You are comforted by the outreach from the farthest reaches of the planet and reminded of the sometime blessings of social media. The accolades came pouring in on the anniversary of her passing and they warmed my heart: -

"Rosie, I see you and hear you on a sunny day as the orange trees are blooming, I remember you when I go to the sea and listen to the waves. Thank you for the wonderful memories …." Almila (her friend in Turkey and the co-founder of the Breast Cancer Awareness group in Antalya.) "Rosie, two days before you left, you called me and said, *thank you Almila, thanks for everything*, even though you were struggling to talk. First time I realized in my life that I would talk to you and not say *see you soon*… you have been and will continue to be such an inspiration to so many and have shown us all how to be positive and how to live life to the fullest.…"

"My life has been richer for your presence and I'm truly proud to have been able to call you my friend. Fly high, Rorabud! I will miss you forever, but you will always be with me in my heart – love you girl!" Sue.

"Love you forever, Rosebud. Please look out for my 17-year-old Barney who just left us one week ago today. He was a naughty cheeky teenager – just like you and me …" (my sister's old friend Bella who just lost her son in a tragic car accident.)

Other friends sent me gifts of photos I had never seen of our girl in full life force from years ago – fun and laughter frozen by time. I want to start compiling all the love and the emotions into a tangible entity for a journey through grief. My Rosie book will be my next project.

When she was passing on two years ago, my husband took me to Salinas River State Beach, where we sprinkled my Mum's ashes years ago. I was in unbearable pain that day, as we knew Rosie's heart was still beating, but that she would never wake up again. It was the gap between life and death I had never experienced before, a road never traveled. Some amazing things happened to me on that beach that day and I felt the urge to pilgrimage – for want of a better word – back to the same place this year. I had also gathered driftwood that day and made my sister a memorial called a 'Rosie Boat' a nod to her love for boat trips and the sea. I knew that we would not be able to give her a traditional send off, since she would be buried the same day in Turkey, as their customs are, but I felt the need to build my own memorial, a place where I could go and talk to her, a place where I had already communed with stunning dragonflies, our shared spirit creature, the day she was leaving the planet. I constructed the Rosie Boat in the Secret Garden next to my mother's urn and by the ponds, surrounded by butterflies, dragonflies, hummingbirds, turtles, water, flowers and peace. I laid special things around the Rosie boat, like a watery grave site, and painted the memorial in different colors and glitter. It was a therapy the like of which I had never immersed myself into before; but I'd recommend to any of you in a similar boat – pun intended.

I wasn't sure if we were going to be able to eat at *The Whole Enchilada* in Moss Landing this year, one of our favorite spots; but they had a great system going and outdoor seating with heaters, so it was only a few minutes before we were seated with drinks and appetizers and enjoying the peace of a meal exercised under strict social distancing guidelines. It really is very pleasant to dine with your companion away from the banter and noise of others – no matter that it took a global pandemic to get us to that place. The crab enchiladas and guacamole did not disappoint our palates, neither did the chilled Morgan Chardonnay. We then took off for the beach. The rest of the world seemed to already be there – plus groups of lovely horses I could watch all day, that were strolling along the sands and snorting into the ether. A feast of water birds – pelicans, cormorants and sea gulls were *helping* the fisherman on the beach and dive bombing into the swell for more. The usual swirly waves of greys, silvers, blues and greens crashed to the shore – rip tide over rip tide. Not an ocean for the elementary bather. Cloudy skies alternating with dark greys and patches of azure made for a superb photographer's palette. I ran the 933 paces from the mouth of the beach to where surely a few sprinkles of my Mum's ashes would still remain (she was born in 1933, hence an easy number to recall!) Away from the mouth of the beach, where most people hang out, the beach becomes quite desolate and, to my mind, even more magical. I start looking for my Rosie boat driftwood and there I find it – a similar color to the original piece but asking for an inscription that I would not hasten to complete. There is no race on the grief journey, no place where you will likely be able to stop after a while and say – 'okay, all done there then!' It is a road well-traveled, but not one we are much good at traversing – a human condition that we will suffer over and over, if we live long enough. I am still just about as bad at navigating grief as I was two years ago, though I cry a little less perhaps. Is that progress? The jury is still out.

Here is the deepest secret nobody knows

(here is the root of the root and the bud of the bud)

And the sky of the sky of a tree called life; which grows higher than soul can hope or mind can hide)

And this is the wonder that's keeping the stars apart

i carry your heart (i carry it in my heart)

--e.e. cummings

(2020)

The New Chair

My poor friend was in bed with a bad back. "Had a busy week?" she asked, thirsty for news outside of her sick bed. "Ack, too busy!" I squealed in return and went on to tell her about my week for the next 30 minutes. Well, she did ask! First, we had our largest fundraiser of the year for the animal rescue – *Pinot For Paws* – a resounding success. Next it was off to the Central Valley for the Celebration of Life for my friend's mother – and all the interesting adventures that come along with that sort of occasion, not to mention the mid-California heats that will sucker-punch you in a micro-second. (Note to self – do not step on the pool concrete in the heat of the day with your naked foot!) Back home again in the more forgiving airs of Monterey County, I did some work, laundry, groceries, animal-related duties. Just sharing my traveler tales from the last few days made me completely exhausted all over again. Gosh, how does anyone have time to read a book anymore, let alone finish the book they are supposed to be working on, or write a story for their weekly column! It's Father's Day weekend and I hadn't even unpacked. Thank goodness, our son canceled his Sunday visit, or I would have had closets packed with dirty laundry and unpacked bags I still couldn't deal with.

Our daughter made it home though – two days prior to Father's Day. And she made it with a plan. A long time ago, she hatched a plot to buy her dad a new reclining chair for his *area*, as we call it. This *area* is a very shabby corner of the family room where he works on his home inspection reports, a place where he snacks, eats and watches tv. Also, sleeps. He pretty much has roots in that corner of the room; even the odd mouse has been known to hang out back there, safely in the knowledge that there will always be things to eat and no danger of any cats entering the toxic zone. When the kids come to visit, they always sink into the nasty old chair, maybe as a sort of primal effort to smell the skin of their father all over themselves again. I would never sit there – it is completely disgusting, as far as I am concerned; but he loved it. The more people would criticize his nasty chair, the more he would beam lovingly and stretch out almost flat with his arms above his head in contented fashion. Even his mother expressed concern that he was increasingly spending the night in the darn thing, but what could you do? It was a sort of indescribable love for a super gross object that completely flawed me, but pretty much ensured I got the whole of the Cal King bed to myself most nights.

"How am I going to get him out of the chair?" my daughter hissed at me, noting that the new chair would be arriving in 30 minutes. "Just tell him!"

I whispered back. We peeked around the corner at this human root vegetable, not looking as if he were going anywhere for the foreseeable future. I slink over, helpfully, towards his corner. "Francoise has something to tell you, dear!" I broached. He sat up sharply, or as much as you can in a recliner with no springs. "Well?" He enquired, just a little more boisterous than usual, glaring at her left hand. That can only be one of two things!" We laughed. "Noooo, dad!" Francoise tittered. "My brothers and I have bought you a new chair for Father's Day and it's arriving in 22 minutes; so, you need to get out of this one!" To our amusement, he didn't seem remotely relieved; honestly more alarmed, if anything.

The beautiful new dark brown leather recliner arrived. We made him go to his man cave outside, while it was being set up in the corner of his area and made to look entirely splendid and welcoming. Eventually he was allowed back in to feast his eyes on his new chair, his new clean space, his new working area. He sat down awkwardly, frowning. "Do you like it, dad?' Francoise broached. Not being, perhaps, the most gracious receiver of gifts on the planet, I was so ready for the standard, flat 'Yeah, it's nice,' response, when I customarily use the dagger-flash of my eyes for tools. "Yes, darling, it's lovely!" he struggled in response, still frowning.

All ready to get the old cesspit chair out of my house and to its proper funeral and final resting place at the local dump, the old man duped my efforts and, instead, steered the ship away from the trash pile and towards the outdoor man cave, or shed, where he proceeded to set it up. "Perfect!" he announces. "I can sit out here as well and do my inspection reports! Just need to run some electric!" Oh my, how we laughed.

The next morning, I get up and the beautiful new chair is on dirty old bricks in our family room, so that it is tilted back at the same angle as the old one. "What the …?" I choke. "It's just not quite right, dear!" He counters quickly. "Needs wearing in, or something …" and, mumbling, off he goes to the man cave to relax in the stinky old one we had done our best to remove, for the collective good, from the household.

We cannot get upset with him, as I relayed cautiously to his rather upset daughter. In 20-years' time, the new chair will be just as *perfect* as the disgusting old one that is now out there in the man cave for the cats to pee on. We just have to accept that he is a stubborn old beast who likes it how he likes it. His mother agreed, noting that he probably got that quality from her. Somehow, I couldn't find argument with that.

(2019)

The Patience Bone

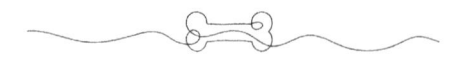

If we have made it to the reading and writing stages of our life, we have all been 4 years old. I asked my husband about his earliest memories; he thinks he was 3. I think I was 3 also, but my 4-year-old memories are really very clear. If you were to ask her, our granddaughter would say she is 4.5. I'm sure her memories are very clear at this stage in her life and level in her development.

Like most modern-day parents, both of her parents are working; one is working and going to school. They are no longer together per se, but they co-parent very successfully. They live in Sacramento; so, it is not easy for either one of them to pop over for the day and bring their child from the city heats to the country breezes. That is where the grand parental unit comes in. Though we are also super busy people in our own right, still both working, plus taking care of the husband's mother and a ranch full of rescues, I told my husband we needed to make it happen. It was our task and responsibility to put some lovely memories into her bank to build on over her formative years. Just seeing her once every 3 months or so, is not enough. And so, the plan was hatched.

"She keeps asking when I can bring her over!" Our son stresses about everything. He royally failed to bring her to see us on Father's Day and she wasn't going to forget that in a hurry. 4.5 year olds don't forget much, I've noticed. And so, we planned to drive to Sacto on July 4th and bring her back to the ranch. It's quite the drive to take in one day, but husband won't leave his mother overnight, and we have no other elder coverage, so there wasn't a choice. Our little girl was so happy to see us; she could hardly stand herself. "3 whole nights and nearly 4 days!" She chirped. Husband and I gulped just a little. After a quick sandwich with the boy, we started the long ride back. "Yes, she still naps!" he said cheerfully, strapping her into her car seat. We imagined that would happen on the journey back and prepare us for her burst of freedom as soon as she hit the ground running at our place. It did not. It also did not happen the entire time she was with us – the full 4 days of her visit. Nor did she go to bed on time. Like at all. It was as if her time with us was, for her, so brief and precious that she didn't want to miss a minute. But she did get extremely tired. And that is when you must dig up the patience bones.

We swam, we played with the animals, we read stories, we selected the kittens she was going to take home, we rode bikes, we swam some more, we picked plums and made jam. We did all measure of fun things that grandchildren should get to do with their grandparents during the summer.

4.5 is a challenging age, I noticed. You do forget, when it's been a while since you had one of those little munchkins under your direct care and supervision for a period of time. They have no fear and when you tell them no, either they do it anyway, or they challenge you with a 'why?' I found the *doing it anyway* concept very frightening, because anything can and does happen on a ranch. The 'why' challenge was fine the first time around, but by about the 3rd why on the same subject your patience wears a little thin. Her patience with us wore a little thin too, when our boundaries were tested time and time again and we had to put our grandparently feet firmly down. At one point her socks and shoes flew across the room in a temper tantrum, when she tired of trying to get them on the right feet. "You have to find your patience bone," I told her. "Where is that?" she responds, still mad and scowling. "Well, it's in there somewhere. You just have to look for it." She looked up and down her arms and legs. "I don't see it," she scowled some more. "No, well I don't either, but you must look for it and then when you find it, use it." I almost immediately realized that the same thing could be said for he and I, golden oldies, in our communication skills with the 4.5 year old politician. Our patience bones also needed retrieving from wherever they had hidden themselves.

"I see why you are always getting in trouble at home," I tell her. "When you challenge the adults in your life and then do whatever it is they don't want you to anyway, you are putting yourself in danger and that means you are being naughty, and you are headed for trouble." She smiled with a glint in her eye. I realized, in her busy world of being shunted from one parent to another and to her Gran's apartment where she spends a lot of her time, she had to find ways to be heard, to be noticed. If she did things she was not supposed to, adults were going to notice her, and her goals would be achieved. There was a kind of mad logic to her behaviors.

We dropped her off with 2 kittens and a bag full of memories – and dirty clothes – at our Santa Nella exchange point, the pea soup restaurant. Sitting in traffic about 10 minutes later, our son took a selfie of her fast asleep in her car seat and sent it to us. "She hit a wall," he tells us. She could no longer refuse to rest or refuse to stop. Her mini-vacation was over and her body was going to steal some delayed slumber and catch up.

I came home to the unreal quietness a little numb, after being the caregiver of a tornado for a few days. I realized that we had indeed had a lovely time together, we had got closer and learned more about each other. We had also tested each other's patience bones on several occasions and we would have to watch that the next time. And I'm not even just talking about the 4.5 year old!

(2019)

The spirits of Thanksgiving past

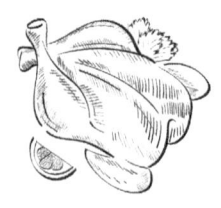

Ah, those memories, like the corner of my mind. Most days we chug along, casting a glance back once in a while when Facebook reminds us of something, or if it's Mama's birthday and she's no longer of the planet – or it's sister Rosie's anniversary and I need to again make the time to fix up her Rosie boat memorial in the Secret Garden. You can get nudges from Saint Elsewhere quite often if you are open to receiving them.

But there is nothing like a mega holiday, like Thanksgiving, to put you in your place and remind you of where you are in life. You never forget the folks who didn't get to come to dinner this year, the ones who chose not to make it for some painful reason or those who are residing just a step away from being able to do that. Someone told me 3 feet off the ground is where you can find that particular essence of spirit, if you are lucky to be indulged by any type of intersection of planets.

If I am hosting Thanksgiving, I like to set an extra place at the table to remind us of those that we are missing. It's a sentimental nod to time, clock of our lives and our hearts, and a barometer of the things that truly matter. The days we speed through life without even casting a glance at memories left in the dust on the wayside; they matter less.

I love Thanksgiving; I've said it before. Not having grown up in the Thanksgiving culture, being – ahem – British at birth, it took me a while to come to the table. But when I came, boy did I. I have learned to love the sweet with the savory (see ambrosia and turkey on the same plate, no less!) I have come to understand that every clan has their own tradition they like to repeat year after year (see weirdly raw broccoli salad, also on the plate with the ham and the turkey, stuffing, gooey sweet hot yams, potatoes and gravy. Also, ambrosia. Still trying to figure out that strange creature we call blancmange in the UK). I'm a creature of tradition; I love it when people hold tight to them year after. I respect that wholeheartedly; whether or not I can actually stomach their tradition on my dinner plate.

I also like the Thanksgiving holiday reminder that the generations roll on like time itself. When I first met my husband, the feasting day was hosted by his mother and father at their home in Freedom. Then his dad passed, and the beacon was slowly, but ceremoniously, passed on to the next generation who brought all the dishes to Mom's house and cooked most of the meal. Then Mom leaves and the next generation takes over. The last few years, we have hosted Thanksgiving at our house with aunts and uncles and his mother. When Aunt Marvel passed on, my daughter took over her tradition of making the devilled eggs. I'm sure she will do that until she passes over the baton to her daughter. You get the idea.

Before you know it, it's time for the generation below you to take over the trusty baton of tradition and run with it. "We are so nervous!" my daughter said. (She and her boyfriend Aaron were hosting the meal at their home we call *The Hacienda* in Arroyo Seco). Though everyone was going to assist – we were bringing ham and sides, his side of the family the same – I understood her nervousness. The baton was being passed down to the next generation and that's a big deal when it happens. The house has to get cleaned, meals planned and prepped – everything has to be just right when the two families are coming together for Feast Day. But it wouldn't be right without the odd dysfunction … the cat has to get out when he's not supposed to, the dog rolls in cow pats and then takes off after you give her a bath and you can't catch her. You didn't quite buy all the things you were supposed to, but it's all fantabulous. Nothing in life is perfect and Thanksgiving Day has a way of reminding you of that. Like life itself, it wouldn't be right if there were not some hiccups along the way.

We arrived early to be helpful to our hosts and calm their nerves. We organized the snack table and made sure everything was on track for when the other half of the clan arrived. The sun was shining, chairs were situated, cushions were turned upside down to give an air of cleanliness and lack of dog hair to the gathering. And, in the end, it was all lovely; it always is. "Aren't you so proud of them?" I asked the other side, as the meal with all its parts came together. He said he was. Grandma and grandpa were there too from Montana, so now we had multi-generations gathering together. Summer sausage, townhouse crackers and cheese balls were served at the snack table in case any of us might forget where we came from. Memories sometimes come from the funniest places. Too bad our granddaughter couldn't have made the melee from Sacramento to add an 8-year-old buzz to the mix, but it had to be amazing just as it was. All the food came out amazingly well, the conversation was fun and engaged and I saw lots of happy faces that day. Early Christmas gifts came out in plastic bags, and I just had to have a really good giggle at that.

When everyone left and it was time to watch the 49er game on the big screen outside on the patio under the stars, I just had to invent a new tradition of my very own. If my daughter was going to be hosting Thanksgiving at her place, then I would be staying right there with her. Give a woman some borrowed jammies and the loan of a toothbrush and you've created something new. And how perfect was that! We even managed to sneak in some *National Lampoon's Christmas Family Vacation* to put the Dysfunctional back into the Functional on a holiday that will live on in our memories, even though we forgot to take any pictures. Our memories will just have to stay framed in those special moments the way some memories are.

(2023)

Travels with Father

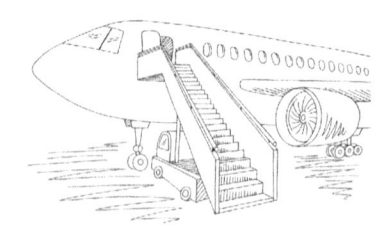

I knew it couldn't be easy; wouldn't be easy. He was over 90 and didn't travel well, hadn't for years. However, he wanted me to take him to stay with my sister for Christmas on the Isle of Man in the middle of the Irish Sea. He's my father and aged over 90. How do you say no? I obviously couldn't. I braced myself. I told him I wasn't going to get upset with him that day.

We were both ready nice and early and waiting for the cab, as our family invariably does. He then calls and tell them to come early anyway – we were ready already. Off we go. All is well. We arrive at the London City Airport and there are busy holiday travelers milling round everywhere. All these throngs of people are making me nervous. I am in charge of the luggage cart, but it feels as if I should be guarding the father, strolling intrepidly ahead with his one walking stick. Clearly no one else was paying attention to him. In a freeze-frame that you keep re-living and cannot lose from the mind, he trips up the kerb, and face-plants squarely on the concrete in front of the airport. I still have not quit reliving that moment. I saw our Christmas holiday melt away in a mesh of emergency rooms and broken bones. He turns over and the blood is all over his face. People flock around to help him up and I feel wildly out of control. 'Ok dad, I'm here, I'm here," is all I can meekly manage as I struggle to reach him through the melee and not lose entire contact with all our assets on the luggage cart. Kindly bystanders help him up and I'm momentarily wondering if that was a good thing to do, but too late; it all happened so fast. The First Aid Wheelchair arrives, father has blood streaming down his face. "I don't want any fuss," he says. "We need to go and check in." At this point I have to get firm and tell him that we are not going to be able to check in with blood streaming down his face. The first aid gentleman is patient and kind and cleans him up. "Don't contact your sister!" he tells me. More pressure. She will be picking us up at the other end and she will not have the heads up she needs to be able to deal with this type of messy arrival.

We land safely, we are safe, no further drama, no broken bones. She is there to greet us and thank God for that. There is a lot to be said for shared sibling-parenting. As she greeted me, I whispered the warning "Face-plant. He face-planted at London City." He then proceeded to tell her all about it. She accommodated with the ice and the inflammatories and the raised leg situation as soon as we got back to her house. He was shocked and bruised, but he was not remotely broken, and we were so glad for that. The following day he was still bruised and sore, also traumatized, but with no serious damage done. Christmas came and we were able to celebrate so nicely. Sister ordered a wheelchair to assist with our outings and we were able to go and visit our other sister's bench, constructed in her memory. Though father insisted on bossing her around over the *boulders* and navigating the generally rough terrain in his wheeled chariot, we safely arrived at our sister's memorial bench with no fights or injuries, and that was a special time.

From then on, we would load up the wheelchair, unload the wheelchair and father would stroll on ahead while we were left back there with the wheelchair, trying to catch him up. We did have to laugh at that. 90 or not, he remained stubborn and spirited, and we had to admire him for his continued quest to be independent. There was even a priceless time when sister was pushing the wheelchair, father was walking without the wheelchair, father noted he would need the wheelchair cushion if he was going to sit in it, sister runs back in the cold rain to get it, positions the cushion in said chair and father still refuses to sit in the chair. Oh god how we laughed.

There are times in life when you can really appreciate your siblings, especially when you are sharing the ornery stubbornness of your ageing parent. I cannot imagine how it would be to deal with this type of stuff as an only child.

As we were leaving sister's home to return back to father's house in London, I was a bit nervous. We had not arrived in an easy way. He was already starting to work himself up into a lather at the prospect of traveling back home. I tried to stay calm, I told him I wasn't going to get upset with him that day. (Part 2). I knew it was going to be a long day; the day I needed to get him home safely. "You have one job, sister," my sister wags at me. "Just one job." And I knew what she was telling me. Just get father home safely with no blood or drama. Just that one job. Her raised eyebrows told me that she knew that was not an easy ask.

He was already shaking before we even checked in our bags. He would not allow any assistance. There was standing and waiting involved; but still no assistance was required. We were 15 minutes late taking off; he couldn't fathom the delay. My head was pounding. I would not get upset with him today. I sipped on my tea onboard and did my breathing exercises. We landed safely and I felt things start to calm a little, until luggage retrieval which is always a little stressy. Fortunately, our cabbie was waiting for us, and it was a cabbie he knew. The cabbie was allowed to push the luggage cart and he, surprisingly, took my arm as we walked towards the cab. Thank gawd, I thought to just myself. I can now get him safely into the car where he will be able to relax. (*One job, just one job, sister*, I hear her say and I hope I can accomplish at least that one job.)

In the cab at last and he's chatting away without a care in the world, happily chomping away on his lunchtime sandwich. Meanwhile I am sitting in the back of the cab with a pounding head and a little ticky eye that seems to have a mind of its own. We finally make it back to his house and I soon escaped, the tension and pressure still reminding me of the last few hours that were.

Last thing I heard was I did such a fabulous job that he wants me to take him back to sister's for his 91st birthday. Oh my.

(2020)

Visiting in situ

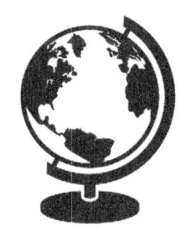

In my newfound practice of giving people an experience instead of a gift, it was going to be our oldest son's birthday and he was no longer going to be receiving socks and underwears from us, or even a normally coveted plaid shirt. I caught wind of the fact that he liked the band Duran Duran – an old English 80's band and thought how fun would that be! The band was going to play in Sacramento shortly after his actual birthday, and this would give us an excuse to head up there and visit with the fam, as well as get to enjoy his birthday gift with him. Those are the best kind of presents! His girlfriend confirmed that that would be a super awesome birthday celebration and he would so love it. Though I've always considered him a bit more of a heavy metal or punk rocker than an 80's hair band, I was thrilled to think I could also catch a show I had missed a mere 40 plus years ago and experience it with him. He received the tickets on his birthday and was "super stoked" about them. So much better than socks and undies! We realize that these young folk are in the crazy times of their lives, building their careers, raising their kids … they don't have much time to come and see their old parents, so we must make the effort to go and see them. "It's important to come and see you in situ," my dad used to say, and he and Mum religiously came over from England twice a year to do just that. I get it now. These days, we are the ones that need to make the extra effort – that older generation. We are them.

Time flew by, as it does during a busy summer season full of visitors coming and going. We hadn't seen our oldest and his family all summer, despite his repeated assertions that they were going to take some time off and come down. But soon it was time to prepare for showtime, the late celebration of his birthday. Since the concert also coincided with our 25th wedding anniversary – ahem – we were going to head up there and have dinner at his swanky restaurant the first night and then go to the concert the following evening.

After a horrendous journey via the gnarly 680 to our destination in Rocklin, we had about 5 minutes to primp for dinner and head out again. And what a dinner it was! Our son is the Director of Wine, and his lady is front end manager at Hawk's Restaurant in Granite Bay, and, for a change, he and his lady had the evening off and were joining us for dinner. Their crew did such a marvelous job of spoiling us at every turn. Our granddaughter joined us, and the feast included – for her, salad and chicken tenders – and for us gnocchi, halibut, black cod, duck confit and much more. A real delight for the senses! Naturally, our son beautifully paired each course with some delicious wines, and we felt so very spoilt, closing down dinner and the restaurant with a fabulous, tummy-warming sherry. We remarked on our way home how lovely it is when you can hang out with your adult children and enjoy each other's company. It can be a long slog through the teens and 20's, but when you get to that happy day, it is truly angels that are singing in your heart. The following day was peace and quiet, pool day and slumber in our air-conditioned room. We had to prepare ourselves for the concert night ahead which was going to be a late one. We barbecued steaks at Marc's house in Citrus Heights and enjoyed some discussions about real estate and the possibility of them moving to a larger home – exciting growth adventures ahead. Then it was game day. We got an Uber to the Golden 1 concert venue downtown and joined the throngs of 80's enthusiasts. Casing the room full of 80's memorabilia, we felt strangely young.

What a fabulous show they put on and all the same original band members seemed to really enjoy themselves, which is not bad for a group that has been playing together for about 40 something years! My heart was very full when we left the concert and my soul full of timeless music. Another of many concerts under my belt and another reminder that I need to write up my 40 something years of concert going and all the epic stars I have seen in my lifetime with, hopefully, more still to come.

It was nice to come back home after such a satisfying visit. We were a bit tired and very full of good food and fun. "We have to make a plan to visit every 3 months and see them in situ," I say to husband. "We must make the effort, so that we stay in touch with their lives and the development of our granddaughter. When Madison is a teen, she will want little or nothing to do with us. She's 8. Now is the time." With that, I started researching something fun to do with her for her 9th birthday celebration up in Sacramento. I was channeling my dad, and also remembering my grandparents and all the efforts they made to come and see us in situ, as it were. Though I was only 9 myself when my grandpa died, I remember him so fondly. The vinyl records and record player he bought for me, the love he showed. I can recall the chocolate frosting on grandma's chocolate cakes and the fact they used to be fine with us bouncing on their enormous bed in the pink spare room and causing all kinds of chaos. A glorious hotspotch medley of memories – all good ones.

As we traverse through this sometimes-crazy life, take time to dwell on the good stuff – the happy visits with your kids and grandkids, the pleasures of good food and music, the trips to go and see your people in situ, where you can once again count all your blessings. We did that last week.

(2023)

What becomes of a broken heart?

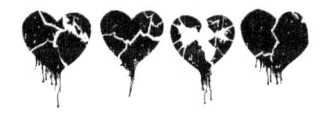

What does become of a broken heart? In the olden days, when romantic liaisons fell apart, ladies would return home quietly to lick their wounds in private, take care of elderly relatives, or forever wear black, in mourning for the life they had wanted and lost. They would sink quietly into the shadows of life, ('Better to have loved and lost, than never to have loved at all.') Forever scarred, they might as well be widows. Nowadays, the young ladies, having fallen off the horse, get right back on it.

My daughter moved down to Shell Beach to start her new life a few years ago and she made a heck of a go of it – new job, friends, apartment, boyfriend. She introduced us and all our friends to a lovely part of the world we had never known before. We thought she was all set and going to be there forever; but forever is a very long time and things fell apart with the boyfriend; she also hated her job. She could have fixed the job situation; the other not so much.

Before we knew it, she was coming home again. I remember very clearly how difficult it is to return home once you have left, especially after a good chunk of time like that. I had to do the same thing many years ago with my parents and I distinctly recall how tricky it was to be back there in that house with those people. I loved them very much, but I did not want to live with them anymore. Those were tricky days – my mother asking me if I would be back in for dinner, my father asking me awkward questions about my future plans.

It was just dreadful going backwards in life like that, and I didn't stay long. But those things can change too, and, in modern times, it is very difficult for young people to live by themselves; so, returning home is not such an unusual event, if only for a little while. Home is a place to take stock, regroup, enjoy home-cooked food, do laundry without needing coins, and think about what is next. It's a precious safe haven when you need it, as many of us do in the ladder of life.

We rescued our daughter and her belongings from Shell Beach, dragging a cumbersome trailer behind us as we returned north again. Her dad had told her previously that he wouldn't be moving her again – and he chose to remind her of this on our journey home – and here we were. He got a mouthful from me for that. She cried all the way home and for days after. Then the light came on; she was tired of crying, and she realized that boyfriend was not really the man she had wanted him to be. She was more grieving the life she had wanted to have, than the one she actually did. She had also adored her apartment near the water. I told her that was just geography; in time, she could recreate whatever pieces of that life made her happy.

She went on to reconnect with old friends and do some fun things. The two of us went for a run around the Bay and ate clam chowder on the wharf. She got her old job back and caught up on her sleep. These were not the days she had planned for herself, but these were the ones she needed, apparently. She helped her Mum out with poor old sick dad and started to clean out the closets and clear cabinets in the home. It started to appear that everything does happen for a reason. She had not planned on returning to her childhood house – we had not known she was going to need to; but here she was, and we were ultimately so very happy to have her back with us, diluting the difficult times we were having all by ourselves and adding an extra layer of nursing care and ability to the mix. We needed the help, and she needed the port in the storm – and what a wonderfully symbiotic combination that can be, when the time is right.

What becomes of a broken heart in modern times is that you return home to heal. You find your peaceful place with the ones that truly love you and you take the time you need to come back to and rebuild yourself. When you are in your mid 20's, it is never easy to come back to someone else's house and pick up where you left off, because you are not the same person anymore and neither is the place you left behind. But this is what reminds you that good family is the backbone in your life with eternal bonds of support that make you who you are.

I have a feeling our girl is going to be just fine. She will find herself again, she will be stronger and wiser for all her experiences, and she will, ultimately, be able to move on and out into the world much better able to cope. For our part, our house will likely be a lot cleaner when she leaves again, our possessions nicely culled and her dad on his way back to good health. These are reasons to be cheerful. Her damaged heart will heal, and her spirits rise. She will come to understand that the road she was on was not the one the universe had planned for her. I told her not to be sad that it is over, but to be happy that it happened. That's what my fabulous Granny Myrtle told me on more than one occasion, having lost 3 husbands in her life, plus a crossroads where she nearly married the 4th, before he too keeled.

Life is one long journey full of colorful pictures, events and people. Seldom do the same images and characters ride you through to the very end. "I thought we'd be together forever," she cried to me. I reminded her that forever was a very long time and most of us don't ever get there.

(2020)

Young love

Her Mama was the first of my friends to get pregnant – it was a strange time for all of us, not least her! She gave birth to a healthy baby girl, named Jessica Starlight. Plump with blue eyes and blond hair, she really was the most adorable little doll. Years on and little Jessica was a grown woman and getting married. That beautiful baby had blossomed into a confident young lady who had found herself a wonderful man and they had already bought their first home where they happily lived with their cat Chester. That is how time flies. These days we seldom get invited to weddings, mostly funerals. But now our children are getting married and how fabulous is that! Life canters along in her inimitable way.

Somehow Jess' mother's oldest friends managed to cadge invites to this spectacular affair, on the Kent Coast of England in a classic old seaside hotel where her grandparents had married 60 years ago; and how excited were we! It was one of those *well, you have to be there* events, never mind I reside on the West Coast of America! A bit like a class reunion, if you like. A group of us schoolfriends for over 40 years gathered there on the Thursday for the meet and greet banquet. Our room boasted a splendid sea view and comfortable accommodations, somehow right next to the bridal suite. I felt like a very lucky girl.

The night before affair was a scrummy buffet dinner, an air of excitement from both families in the air. Toasts and speeches flowed like the wine. Many people had traveled in from abroad, like me. Families and friends gathered together, as you only really can at either weddings or funerals. Cousins raced up and down the impressive staircases. My friend and I decided we needed some fresh air and went off on a stroll along the promenade after dinner. All of a sudden, the impulse took us that we needed to indulge in a night swim in the millpond of a sea before us, with the moon guiding our path into the flat black water, so we stripped off, as you do when you are 55 and nobody cares and ran into the water. A wily mama cormorant kept watch over us on her nest in the groin over the sea. Spirits zoomed around us overhead. It was a wonderfully special night. We eventually dripped our way back into the hotel, bumping into other wedding revelers who also thought that a night swim was a marvelous idea, and soon everyone was headed back out to the beach for a night swim, the air full of excited young ones squealing with joy. I think we actually enjoyed 3 swims that night.

The next day was wedding time. The bride and her sister were beautified in the wedding suite with the door on the latch, so anyone – save the groom – could pop in and see what was going on. There was so much love in the room. The Ceremony itself took place in the same ballroom where her grandparents had married 6 decades before, overlooking the beautiful sea. When the bride appeared on the arm of her father, there were lots of teary eyes in the rows. I caught the look of her husband to be, overcome with love as she arrived by his side, and I felt so happy for them.

The sun shone fabulously for all that entire afternoon. The wedding breakfast was a fun, cheerful affair with delicious food. Later on, it was boogie time, and the dance floor was filled with the 55-year-olds grooving their little hearts away, as if they hadn't done that in quite a while; and maybe we hadn't! Lots of photos were taken that day and night – divine frozen moments of love and happiness. My heart was very full.

The next day was time to pack up and leave. Everyone's finery was put away. I felt oddly numb and tired as if I had witnessed a very special event that I would want to process later and enjoy on the darker days. I sent over my snap shots and videos I had captured so others could enjoy the frozen moments also.

Now we are of an age that our children are getting married and having children, it is so heartwarming to remember the beauty of young love, the passion and enthusiasm of young ones just getting started in life from your armchair of wisdom and experience several decades ahead. "All we want is for our children to be happy', us golden oldies noted to one another and it's a pretty simple thing. Except it's not. Marriage requires hard work, great communication skills and the will to try and keep things fresh and exciting. The key to a long marriage is likely a sense of humor – we all agreed that. Long after the passion cools, the humor can keep everything ticking along nicely and the home fires burning.

Wishing Jess and Tom a life full of love, health and happiness … oh and lots of humor, can't forget that.

(2019)

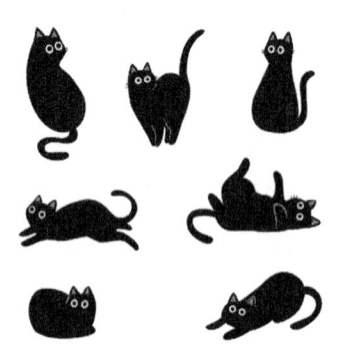

SECTION 2

Me & The Animals

Introduction to – Me & The Animals

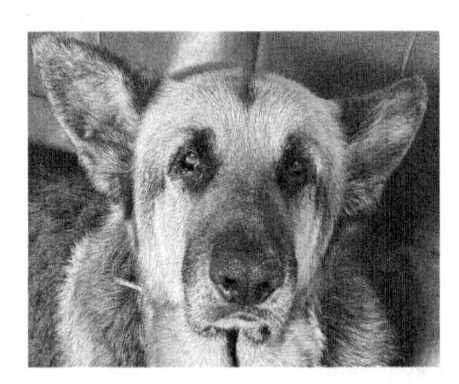

If you know me and my weekly column *Window on the World* in the local papers, you will know how much of an animal lover I am. I was the co-founder of South County Animal Rescue (SCAR) in January 2016, a charity that has grown from strength to strength over the years and one that had its infancy in picking up stray dogs from South County roads and not knowing what to do with them. We have all come a long way since then and I am so proud of the organization full to the brim with Animal Champions and all their amazing work.

The stories in this section are not only about rescue animals, but also some of the madness you bring to your home when you are an animal rescuer. From agreeing to foster two cats that belonged to a stranger for a whole year (and one was a complete terrorist) to reluctantly accepting to foster my first German Shepherd, in order that he not be euthanized. Then falling so in love with him I had to adopt him. Yes, that kind of madness.

But life with the animals is equally rewarding. The unconditional love they give you is one of the most marvelous things you can experience in life. Every time you leave the room – normally they follow you – but, if not, they are always so happy to see you when you walk back in. Look for that kind of devotion from a human! Animal rescue has good and very bad days and that can take its toll on a person; but if we all do a little more than our comfort zone, contribute a little more, foster a little more, participate a little more – then leaps and bounds could be made in our small communities that have already seen enormous progress in the homing of neglected animals and the education of our people.

If you would like to contribute to this incredible charity, please go to scar.pet to find out how, or send me an email and I can guide you. As their founder, SCAR gets all my spare cash and a permanent piece of my heart. Be a part of the change you wish to see.

lucymasonjensen@gmail.com

A year with foster cats

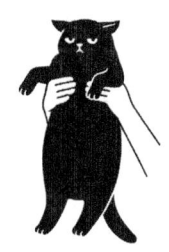

As I may have mentioned before, social media is really good for animal stuff – not so great with some of the other. Just over a year ago, I see a posting that has been shared and shared. This family is in the Bay area and leaving to South America for a year. They have 2 cats that they are trying to find a safe haven for until they return home. They asked friends and relatives – that was a no. They looked at boarding kennels. Wow. They even looked into what it would take to have the cats go with them on their travels. Not an easy task. So, they were looking for help from the animal peeps community, which is rather large, and a royally sharing bunch. My heart was touched that a family would love their pets so much that they would seek to find a foster home for a whole year – that is quite an ask. I contacted Kevin and told him we would take them in, if none of their people could. He seemed surprised and then confirmed that none of his people were willing to take them. I couldn't help but feel a bit snarly that no one close to them would take in their beloved pets, but that's people for you.

Kevin, his wife and two boys arrived with Shadow and Soleil and their possessions. We signed a contract and he agreed to furnish food and supplies for the year. How hard could it be? Soleil spent most of the first week under the bed, quietly getting used to her surroundings. Shadow immediately jumped up onto the counter and began creating havoc. "Ah, newsflash!" I thought to just myself. I'm seeing a little bit why no one wanted to take in this naughty cat for a whole year; but I was fairly used to counter jumpers in my time as a cat lady and shoved him off. Eventually he would tire of it.

We had family over and pizza for dinner. Shadow proceeded to fly through the air and extricate an entire slice of pizza out of my daughters-in-law's hand and took off with it. I had never seen the like! From then on, regardless of how much cat food was available for him to eat, that naughty black cat would pounce on any human food in his view shed and swiftly demolish. Husband's morning bagel and cream cheese – easy-peasy. Someone trying to foolishly have a peaceful lunch up at the bar … gone!

I got Kevin's permission to take him to the vet. Something must be seriously wrong with him if he's always so starving hungry! Several tests later and, no, nothing seriously wrong. They dewormed him, gave him some probiotics. Same behavior. He was just a very, very naughty cat.

Birds would scream and dive at him when he went outside (there was absolutely no way I could tolerate having him indoors all the time like his sister!) He'd ignore them and promptly devour one of their crew in a New York second, enjoying his feast on the lawn right by their nest. Such boldness! "I like him!" My friend observed when she was staying with us. "He's a survivor!"

Oh yes, that he is. A pain in the tush survivor. "You wouldn't like him that much if he was staying with you for a whole year." I respond, not kidding at all. Open a door and he's through the middle of your legs and flying up to a table or countertop where there might be food lurking. Then you can't catch him because he's as swift as a black tornado. "Ooooooh!" I would get so exasperated trying to keep him out of the house when he wanted in. Somehow, he knew when our mealtimes were and that was the funnest part of his day.

He also trained the non-cat loving dogs to respect him, or his claws would come out and he would mercilessly slash them around the muzzle. He could be seen waiting around the corner for an innocent and unsuspecting canine to pass by and be under attack from the feline militia in the household. They won't miss him either.

So, Shadow and Soleil will be leaving us and returning to the arms of their devoted family at the end of the month. I imagine that Soleil will be right back under a bed for a while, civilized creature that she is. And the black monster will be headed for any dinner plate or surface where he reckons he can steal whatever he wants, like the Artful Dodger. "I'm going to miss Grey Cat," (Soleil) pronounced husband a little mournfully. Well, it's a package deal and a contract and the pair of them need to return home, I say. Just as well there is a feral cat that is swiftly becoming non-feral at my office, and he looks like a beautiful lynx. He might well be a sweet bed companion for husband once Soleil goes home.

Will I foster for a whole year again, will I ever foster some one's critters when I know that everyone else has turned them down? That's a very good question. I think the long-term foster thing is way too hard and taking in cats for a year is borderline insane. But we did it, we kept them alive for a year plus and their family has pledged to come and rescue them back from us.

I will never forget my year with Shadow, the black devil – and I say that completely without affection – nor his antics that reminded me how little cats care about your feelings or, apparently delusional, entitlements. They have no manners and no conscience. As for the birds in my neighborhood, I'm sure they will all be cawing with joy when the car finally drives off with their nemesis nicely tucked away in his pink crate making his strange hawk noise and sniffing in the air for any snacks that might be hiding in the car, so he can break out of his locked box and get them.

I will not forget Shadow, but I won't miss him either. It will be nice to have pizza with the family without wondering where he's lurking and waiting to attack. What a year it has been!

(2023)

Be kind to one another

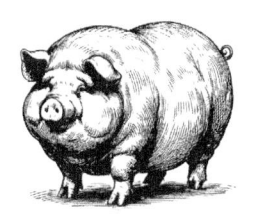

Be kind to one another. 5 simple words that you can hear every afternoon at the end of the Ellen De Generes show. As a working person, I rarely catch the show; but love it when I do. It's such a buoyant and uplifting program. And these are some powerful words. To me, they are the essence of humanity; the goal we humans should have all day and every day of our lives – all of us. If you cannot do at least that, then what are you good for? What are we all good for? If some one is short a dime or a dollar at the grocery checkout, give it to that poor person quietly, without a big old pomp and circumstance, skip the beneficent gesture of 'look at me, how generous am I?' Just do it. It's the right thing to do. If another person needs assistance with their vet bills, or someone needs a ride to the doctor; could you manage that? Many of us could. Do we? Hmmm. Make a difference where you can in the world and some practice that – not just in the pulpits of organized religion, but in the streets where we live, the businesses we frequent, the souls that really, truly need our help. For some, it's a habit that has become a lifestyle and I wish more people practiced it in their every day. The world would be a much better place for it – and that is no cliché. Am I preaching to the choir? I know there are lots of good, generous folk all over the place. We just need more.

For those of you who know me, you could never say I am a political or religious animal. I think those two entities are the biggest dividers in life and, actually, in proven history. To coin a modern phrase, I don't go there; never have, never will. But the harsh reality of modern times does not just pass me by. I absorb it as much as any other person that pays a modicum of attention to the world and her sometime cruel ways; whoever you want to blame – and I don't go there either.

The only way I can get my head around it is, like Ellen, but in a much smaller way, to spread a little joy – that's all the power I have. Recently my chief llama Harold Malcolm Democracy started relaxing on the deck next to my house. Rescued from a llama farm in Nevada, he's lived here with us and his two brothers for around 7 years now and this is a new thing. When his friend, our beautiful horse Sir Winston White Horse, left this planet, Harold's daily mission was to get as close to us as possible, no matter what; as if his friend had told him, 'Take care of those two … they're going to take a little managing without me!' And boy was he right! Harold siddles up to the sliding door of the house and peers into our family room at least twice a day. We think he is looking for Winston, imagining that the large canvas photo we showed him once was actually our horse himself and he's still waiting for him to come out and play. It will not surprise me if he makes it through the living room door one of these days and proceeds to kick back and relax on the sofa. So, what do I do with all this wonder? I share these rather remarkable, often funny, photos of my llama on social media. People chuckle, they laugh, they comment how the llama made their day and turned things around for them in that moment. How could you halt that kind of a response to a simple llama photo? Spread the love. Be kind to one another. None of us really know what the others are going through. It's only a small thing, but it's worth doing if it provides cheer to others.

As the horrors continue in our world, I post a family portrait of my rescue dogs, naturally not lined up as you would want, because, let's face it, they are dogs; but they are there, all together, all the same, in that moment. 'Family portrait time!" I say. "Only 20 canine paws remaining!" (In the last 3 months, we have lost 12!) And instead of echoing anything out in the world that is actually on people's minds and the spouting of the thoughts and prayers that many are doing, paying lip service to awful tragedy upon tragedy in our nation, I simply post a photo of 5 amazing rescue dogs, all sitting sort-of sweetly together and figuring things out. That is the only response I can have. And it seems to help cheer people along. Who knows; maybe they will decide to post a picture of their guinea pig or donkey and delight their world just a little themselves. We could start a movement.

This week, my neighbor picked up a starving, milk-filled Mama Pitt from Metz Road near our homes. Poor baby had her nails and pads worn down and looked as if she didn't have much longer to struggle out there in this world. I have never seen a more hungry or thirsty creature. My husband and I took her back down to the road where she was found, thinking there may be needy puppies somewhere out there in the wilderness, but we didn't find any. Such a sweet girl. Who would do that? Did someone sell the pups and dump her? Did you drive past an animal in need and not stop? Were you busy and couldn't make the time? Could you have called some one else to go out there and save a life? Only you know the answers to that. Ruby, as we called her, will survive and we will make sure that she thrives. Thanks to my neighbor who took the time to stop and pick her up and to the others out there, who salute the posting of the simple animal photos and the hurrah for other pure and lovely things that come across your viewshed. Pass it along. Be kinder to one another. Way kinder than you need to be. It's a nut house out there and often-times, trust me, it is the animals that show us the way.

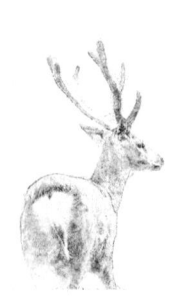

(2019)

Destiny arrives in funny ways

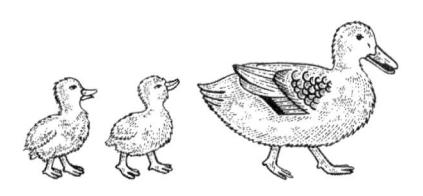

I nearly broke into tiny irreparable shards, when there was nothing more we could do to help him and my horse was finally laid down to his eternal sleep at Solace. It was April 2, 2019, early in the morning. As the strong medicine filled his veins and he fell to the ground, I will never forget the look of peace on his face, his hooves in running position and face raised to the streaming sun. Since I could not bear for him to permanently leave, I had his body cremated so that he would always be with me, (also sprinkled in all the places that he so loved), in a large box in my living room. Naturally his spirit was still everywhere, but regardless, I was inconsolable for a very long time. I pledged that I would never again have a horse in my meadow, the pain was too much to bear when it became time to say goodbye. When you love big, you fall hard, and this no longer surprises. 'Normal' people could not believe how I grieved over my best friend. He had seen me through such tough days. We had learned to trust one another so intensely I thought he might be the one that gets to live longer, and I would need to go first; like an old married couple.

A year ago, the neighbor across the street with his mini ranchita, brought a horse to his meadow that hugely resembled my dearly beloved. When I first caught sight of the flea-bitten grey, I had to pull over the car and take a picture. It was uncanny. Over the past several months, I would look for her every time I drove past. I'd linger at the curve in the bend, checking to see if she had food and water. The ranchita dude was not the best caretaker of such an impressive beast – or, truthfully, any animal. I had rescued my dog Winston Junior from there the day Winston Senior died. Junior had been dumped with a broken leg and left to be eaten by a pack of coyotes. He's now doing fine. Then I rescued my pig, Sally, from there also. She was a victim of pure neglect, also meanness for sure. Was I going to have to rescue this horse also? I had pledged there would be no more horses at Solace. Was I going to break my own promise?

My neighbor and I would take turns in checking on the mare. One furiously hot day in high summer, I just had a feeling the dude hadn't been by. I called the landlord to the property and told him that the animals needed a well-check, and I was going to have to break the lock to the gate. He was fine with that. We went into the meadow and, sure enough, the animals had no food or water. I was so furious. This was the beginning of regular welfare checks on the animals there that included chickens, a dog and horses. The place was ramshackle with broken glass everywhere. The ranchita dude must have heard on the grapevine that there was a livid Brit on the property and swiftly headed over to where we were busy filling up the water troughs for the thirsty creatures. We had also got pet food and hay from Solace to fill their empty bellies. Fortunately, my husband was there, or this guy would likely have received more than just the benefit of my sharp and furious tongue. In short, he asked for a second chance. I consulted my vet and she said that that is what animal control would grant, if asked. He was given this second chance that he did not deserve and rapidly failed the test.

My neighbors and I rallied to save these animals from this diabolical situation and the ranchita dude finally released them to us, naturally at a considerable cost. We bought hay for the horses and started to work on gaining trust long lost. I kept hoping that the flea-bitten grey would find a fabulous home that wouldn't require mine, as her colt did and the other grey with her and the appaloosa earlier. It didn't happen. I would watch her all on her lonesome in my neighbor's meadow. She would be anxiously car-watching and hoping that today she would be able to eat, the same as yesterday. There's nothing like an animal that is insecure about food. Most of my rescues are that way, Winston Senior certainly was, and it is a sad sight to behold.

I would go over there and chat to her and brush her. She was sweet with old-soul eyes and a few war wounds on her legs. She looked so like my boy. She had certainly had her colt in the vineyard when she had broken out of her pen one night in terror and delivered the baby all alone amongst the vines. The vineyard workers had called one of our neighbors and she had been found and returned in a horrible mess. Fortunately, there was no lasting damage done to her or her colt. No thanks to the ranchita dude. I tustled with the decision about what to do.

My boy Winston came to me in a dream and told me it was fine. The mare needed us, and she should make her home here, as he did and his large spirit does – and so many other animals before. And so it was that we decided she deserved a better life among the lost and found souls at Solace. We were going to pay the price asked and bring her home.

She is now safely nestled in Winston's former stable, surrounded by all the abandoned souls that also found their eternal homes at Solace. And this is what we do. Rescue and love the unwanted and restore hope to the hopeless.

"Our farm is finally full!" The husband announced gleefully, and I realized what he meant. The missing gap had been filled. The universe had aligned to make it so. I made a mental note that we had also added 2 turtles, one very large dog and a beautiful mare in the space of less than a month: but who's counting.

When we first started South County Animal Rescue in 2016, it was because the need was so huge and the resources so slim in our area. Not much has changed in that regard, except that there are many more Animal Champions out there doing free and difficult work, day and night. Definitely fewer animals are being euthanized and given up on these days; less dogs and cats are having litters. Surely people are learning about animal responsibility, commitment, and husbandry? I'm not so sure about the last part, but we all soldier on in that regard to educate the ignorant and assist those without resources.

For my part, I am so full with delight that Mary the Mare has found her forever home with us. Now I don't have to watch for her every day and wonder whether she's eating and drinking. Now I know, for sure, that she is here with us. She is safe and she is loved. My promise of the past has fallen by the wayside because it needed to. Winston gave his blessing, and all is well with our world.

(2022)

Find your passion

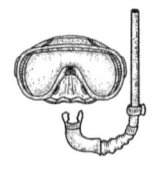

No matter how much you love your work, I have discovered that it is an even more wonderful thing to lead a fulfilling life if you also have passions that you adore, which are disconnected from your employment. Your work life should feed your hobby world; that's how I see it.

My oldest friend and I have been writing the story of our childhoods spent together on the East Coast of England. It has been an epic, rambling journey of digging for old pictures, scanning images, rooting up old memories, laughing all over again (truthfully, we never stop doing that) at our mish mash of memories from 50 plus years ago and then mining deep for some more. For the last several months, this has been our *hobby* of sorts – an infatuation that eats up the hours and has seen me abducting and scanning everyone's photo albums the world over.

My friend Lizzie perhaps never realized what a great writer she is, not to mention a skilled designer and paginator now of the literary world. Maybe this will open new and amazing doors for her in the future! She did the design and layout of my last book, *The Soup Diaries* that I was extremely proud of, and here we are, Project Central all over again. Because Lizzie's mega passion is sailing (like big sailing, not just pootling around a bay) and she has signed up for, not one, but two legs of the Clipper-Round-the-World race, we are under the gun, as it were, to get this book project under our belts, so that she can sail the high seas come January with our childhood project firmly under the proverbial belt.

Of course, my goal is always to have a new book out in time for the *Christmas rush*, but it will definitely not happen this year. *The South Lookout – Our Aldeburgh Childhood* will likely appear in print and kindle – for you non-paper readers – by the end of the year. We couldn't be more excited.

I wish more people read books, I wish more were excited by local authors like me; but then I have to understand that writing and reading are my hobbies, not necessarily others'. "How do you find the time?" Is a question often asked of me. I have a full-on life of other passions including animal rescue, traveling and 49er football, ha ha, plus a little real estate job on the side. I don't watch much television or troll on social media. I make the time because it's my passion. Simply, it fulfills my existence.

"He loves that stupid hunting!" My daughter complains about her boyfriend during duck season. "That's his hobby, his passion. We all need them!" I tell her. "You need to work on your hobbies. Can't be all about the work and the nursing and the school!" (Though I was the same at her age – all about making money and moving ahead in life.)

If you don't have a hobby or three like me, how about finding a cause? That can be just as fulfilling, maybe more so. Back at the end of 2015, when we were mulling over thoughts of forming an animal rescue and organizing what we were already doing, it was the cause in my heart that bred the plan. It took a while to get the plan operational, as it were; and it certainly was not pretty out the gate, but now I look at the charity, South County Animal Rescue, (SCAR), that has become a near household name in these parts; and I am proud to be one of the founders of this incredible cause. My hobby, my passion actually developed into a living, breathing entity that saves lives – and will, I hope, well after I am just a name that is slightly affiliated with it. Too many folk are self-oriented, quiet in their own little worlds of friends and family, that, let's face it, can fill your world quite easily. Add a job into that mix and you may get 7-8 hours sleep a night. But it's not really enough, is it. Could you spare a few hours to volunteer at a soup kitchen, at a school – for your local animal rescue, for crying out loud? You might be surprised how much that can fill your heart, without necessarily sending your daily life into overdrive.

Animal people know how all-consuming rescue life can be. It eats you up because the need is so huge. Perhaps you can solicit some people from your life who are not so busy to be engaged in your cause? Maybe they could foster an animal, help save a life, do something larger than themselves? I cannot tolerate people who are full of their own misery and do nothing for others. There is little purpose in the world with that kind of outlook, in my opinion. We can all do something outside of ourselves to make a difference, enhance a life – maybe even your own.

I have known too many narcissists in my life that just take up space with their own inward-looking eyes. Don't be that. Be part of the solution, the help, the hearts that give not take.

In animal rescue right now, we are in crisis. With the closing of the Salinas Shelter – yeah, it's all about money and budgets and where we can cut now – our County Shelter is over-flowing and faced daily with horrible decisions of who dies next. Did you know that? Perfectly adoptable fur babies are having their lives snuffed out because there is no room at the shelter and no place to put them. Better just to kill them? My culture and nature find that abominable. It hurts my heart every time I see an outreach from the shelter, knowing where this path will lead. What kind of civilized nation are we that allows murder like this? Not civilized at all, if you ask me.

I wish I had a boarding house for all the unwanted. I already have 9 canines at my house – and the mixing of the personalities is a daily challenge I wouldn't wish on anyone. But it's better than the alternative.

If you can't foster for an overflowing shelter, could your mother, brother, daughter? You might be surprised how life-enhancing it is to be a part of the life-saving solution. To be engaged in something outside of yourself.

Please give it some thought and then apply to be a foster parent today at scar.pet. The life you might save may well be your own.

Find your passion. Build a passion. It makes for a much better world.

(2023)

Finding Bruno

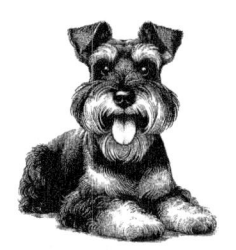

There are so many 'My dog is missing' posts on social media these days, it makes you wonder if all the local dog owners just leave their gates open and hope that their pooch makes it home in time for dinner of an evening. It really is quite astounding. Then I see my friend post that her dog is missing, and she doesn't have any idea how he got out of the back yard. I felt a slight chill go through me. This family is fairly new to town, and they seem like conscientious dog people. How would he have got out of the yard? We started sharing the 'Missing Bruno' post. No sign. They canvas their neighborhood, knock on doors, hang posters. No one had seen this 80lb – give or take – hunk of love. How could he have just vanished? The days pass, and still, he doesn't return home. A reward is offered for his safe return … I hold my breath, still nothing. In rescue work you hear all measure of horror stories about missing animals, and you hope upon hope that this is not the case. As the days compounded, I felt more and more desperate and sad about Bruno's fate. But the sharing upon sharing of the missing pup finally hit upon a lady who thought she had seen him in town. She contacted the family to come over and see and there he was. Skinny and hungry and afraid, but there was Bruno ready to come home. "Did he sleep okay?" I asked, once he was safely home again. "Oh, like a log on top of his human," came back the reply. The family was so overjoyed to have him home and so grateful to their new community for all the help in bringing him home. I was happy to have played a small part in the sharing and sharing among the online community – it really can and does make a difference.

Whether or not you are a fan of social media, it is good for these types of things. The sharing and resharing can have this wonderfully magic compounded effect, so that there is a good chance that some one or thing can and will be found. I was so happy for Bruno and his family I wanted to run over there and hug them all.

It's so lovely to have a story like that with a happy ending. In animal rescue that is not always the case, so we have to take the wonderful ones when we can and hold them tight.

I was also reminded that people are basically good. Ignoring the bad apples that seem to get all the press, most people are kind and want to help. It makes them feel good – it's part of our basic human condition.

"I adopted Chloe from SCAR last year," the lady told me. "My mother had just passed on and Chloe made the world of difference for me. Then my father passed, and I had a little money, and I could think of no better charity to donate to than our very own South County Animal Rescue." I was so gratified that her adoption led to her love and loyalty over the last few years. Also, that a rescue pup would make such a difference in the grieving of a human. But us animal lovers know all about that!

During this season of giving and gratitude, take time to reflect on what has made a huge difference in your life! It is likely not money or a new car, the latest iPhone or gadget. It is likely love – pure and simple – the people around you, the animals that share your life. It's a simple concept, but not really. In the day-to-day madness of our lives, it is easy to bypass the obvious and keep looking ahead at the horizon for bigger and better. Very often what is right in front of us is the most important thing.

If you are looking for something to love, look no further than a rescue animal from your local SCAR. If you have money to give, it's always the season of need at your local animal rescue. You can rest assured that they are all volunteers and none of your hard-earned donations will go towards large salaries or marketing campaigns. Be a part of the change you wish to see in the world. We have learned that through SCAR and it's a wonderful thing to witness.

(2019)

Having babies in your 50's

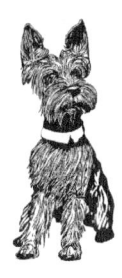

"Why don't we just adopt older dogs from now on. Let's make the end of their lives the best ever!" We were all set. No more puppies, no toddlers with 4-legs. Our pack of near golden oldies (truthfully, more black-and-white than golden) – except for Junior – were spending their last years being beautifully spoiled in the comfort of their peaceful home at Solace.

Move stage forwards. (Not long, I might add.) I get home after a long day. The garage door is unusually shut. I open it and see my husband sitting there with a very tiny black puppy. Oh. My eyebrows rise all by themselves.

"The neighbor honked the horn, I came out. He spoke to me in Spanish, handed over the pup in a bird cage and drove away." "What?" I responded helpfully. "You didn't ask him what the heck, if he found the pup or what?" "He speaks Spanish only and I don't." So, there you had it. A tornado had arrived in the household. Come to find out, after we posted *Found* posters and asked around our neighbors, the dog owner's dog had produced a litter and he wanted to gift us a pup. How nice. A long story about us rescuing his cow Delilah from the vineyard and feeding her for two days without accepting payment in return and then tracking down her rightful owner – and now we get a puppy. That's right. Just what we had said we didn't want.

So, the puppy pads arrive, along with the teething rings, puppy chow, harness and more. You would have thought we had just hosted our own puppy shower. My old collies looked wearily into my eyes, pleading for help as the tiny black pistol pulled at their tails and jumped up on their old bodies. The mean Queen told the whippersnapper where she wasn't welcome, by inserting her head inside his mouth. (He knows better but can't help himself.) Solace had overnight turned into Chaos.

Turd, as she lovingly became known at the beginning of our new adventure, for want of a name we could all agree on, and as animal rescuers the world over acknowledge, if you name the animal you keep the animal, decided that my husband was her human. He was her reason for living, her love absolute. She immediately found her nightly bed in his armpit. You forget what puppies are like. Lights go on at 2am, then 4 and perhaps 5 in your endeavors to potty train the little beast. You are sleep-deprived, and she is just fine. Puppy pads are put down and missed, shoes relocated where they should not be, generally soggy, and then immediately lost again. "Oh, but she's so cute," our daughter pleaded. "If you home her, then I want another puppy." Gawd. We are going on 11 years of living with her grouchy old Queenie and that's all we need. another choice animal for us to raise for her. I had also said no more Queenslands in addition – they are a difficult breed, territorial as a tiger and best in a one dog home. Turd definitely had some Queensland in her, in addition to the very naughty terrorist breed, (terrier) that will cause the other doggies to leave home.

"I'm okay if she gets a really nice family to live with," husband states emphatically. I eyed him cautiously, as the pup leapt up into his lap and lay down in a completely sweet and adoring way. "Well, regardless," "I say. "We have to get her puppy shots done and there's a clinic this Saturday, so I'm taking her over there." I take her along to the clinic, everyone admiring her along the way, and she was so well-behaved in the car I was quite the proud Mama. "What's her name?" the lady asked. "Stella," I replied quickly. "Her name is Stella." Oh heck. I was falling down my own tunnel of places I had been before. If you name, you claim.

"6 is a nice round number!" my friend piped up. "24 canine paws is still a good number. Not like a hoarder at all!" I couldn't argue with that. After all, at one time we were fostering a whole bunch of creatures – 11 dogs to be truthful at the time – and then the Mama dog Molly gave birth to 11 puppies underneath my deck. (You do the math). Husband had to army-crawl under the deck and fish out the newborns. Those were the crazy, insane days of animal rescue. I clearly recall myself telling another friend that I was going to let my golden oldies live out their days and not start adding to the pack until we were down to two dogs again. I lied. Life has a way of giving you whatever it is you are well able to manage and surprising you around the next curve, in our case with a new bundle of love that will likely delight and frustrate us for a good while to come.

My neighbor comes by. "Oh, she is adorable! Lucky you to have got such a beautiful pup!"

"Hmmm," I respond. "The jury is still out as to whether she is staying or not." Then I hear a call from the pond area ... "Linski! Come to Dad!" and off she whizzes. Her fave human was looking for her and that was an immediate call to action.

Stella-Bella-Linski (3 names because we couldn't agree on just one) looks like she will be staying here for a while. At least until she gets through the next two rounds of puppy shots. Oh, and then there will be the rabies shot ... also rattlesnake ...and before you know it, it will be time for her spay. Golly gosh, time flies. I did get her micro-chipped at the shot clinic because that is just the responsible thing to do, regardless of where she ends up. Did I say she travels really well in the car and she only missed 1 of her puppy pads the last two nights? She is learning to be a super ball girl in line with all the other border collies on the ranch and she has also established the pack pecking rights and who not to snuggle up with. Did I say she has the right coloring for our pack – the mottled feet and black and white body of a Collie Champ in a very conveniently small package. Can you tell I am also a little smitten already? Character is fate, as they say.

(2021)

Healing llama karma

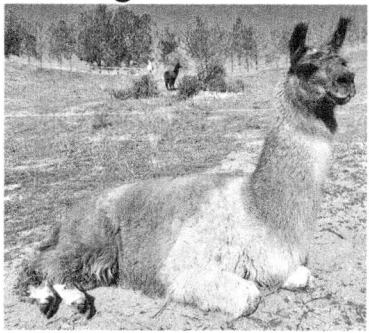

The best made plans, or so they say, are often shot to sugar and this week was no exception. All my January visitors had left, the birthdays were over. It was time to get down to work and taxes – part of my winter lot. I had a beautiful clear week in the diary, ready to get to the tedious business of real life. But then Harold Malcolm Democracy stopped eating. He's my chief llama; if you've never crossed his path before. He is the largest, proudest and most domestic chap amongst my pack of three. This was concerning. It had happened before, but he always came around after a couple of days. I tried to tempt him with all measure of taste treats – his orchard hay and grain, even a little four-way grain that he used to devour. I called on the *Ask Anything Line*, (cost me $5) and, eventually, a llama dude from Nevada tried to help me out. He did have some good ideas. I called my llama lady in Montana who handles Harold's shearing and shots every year. She had some other ideas for him. Nothing worked. He was still not eating, drinking or pooping – as far as I could make out. "They are pretty stoic animals," my llama lady told me. "Once they show you that they are not feeling well, the odds are they are pretty far along in their disease progression." I did not like that response at all. I had lost far too many of my family last year and the year before. I did my own super-vet sleuthing on Google, trying to see if there was anything I hadn't tried. Nope. It was time to bring in the big guns and find a llama vet, of which there are not many locally.

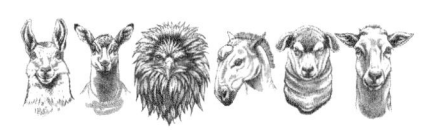

As we do in modern times, instead of going to the near-obsolete phone book for information, we go to social media. I sent a shout out to the world about Harold's condition and asked whether anyone knew a llama vet in these parts. Who knew that our very own local vet claimed to be one of those and so we made a plan for him to come and see Harold. The llama vet admitted to me that not much is known about llamas, and I couldn't have agreed more. If you Google anything about cows or horses, you will never stop finding information. That is not the case with llamas. We put a pony halter on Harold, and he was so well-behaved I was proud of him. He was obviously feeling quite miserable. The llama vet gave him a good going over, took some blood and gave him a couple of shots and, sure enough, he was perky enough to eat some orchard hay the following morning. That gave me reason for optimism. Facebook lit up with happiness when I sent a photo announcement telling them that Harold had perked up and seemed to be eating a little. It made me smile that people that the world over were caring about a big old llama. Always love it when I see a side of humanity to like!

Next day he was off again and seeming to be not in pain, but certainly not improving; again, not eating. My week was rapidly going down the tubes. I was getting little work done and I was worried sick. The llama vet and his trusty assistant returned to try other things on poor old Harold – some of them quite demeaning for a king llama; but he tolerated it all. He knew we were just trying to help him. Friends of mine the world over were also trying to help. Could it be bad grass? Maybe a tooth problem? Ask about hepatic lipidosis! I know ….He's pining for democracy in your country!" One piped up. Oh, dear me. We had the whole litany of Google-ists out there trying to help Harold on his way to feeling better.

The llama vet left us with medicine for him that we will do our best to deliver intravenously, as prompted. This morning he finally came up from the meadow and had a little nibble on some grass and then strolled back down to have another nibble on the ground cover. Dare I be cautiously optimistic that we have finally turned a corner in this strangest of strange llama viruses that no one seems to understand? There is, indeed, much that still needs to be discovered about the beautiful llama. I urged my vet to become the area expert and use my pack for his investigations.

The jury is still out about Harold Malcolm Democracy, but if love can be a cure, then, surely, he will soon be well again, and I can knuckle down to everything I didn't accomplish in the lost week my llama got sick. I remain one very concerned Llama Mama.

(2019)

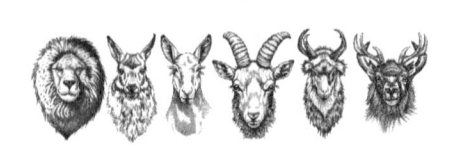

My pumpkin coffee table

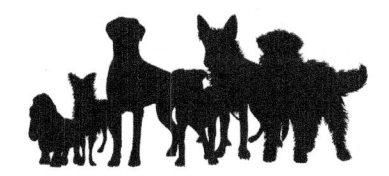

It was the time of our daughter's 8th grade trip with Main Street Middle School to Washington D.C that he was dumped at the gates to our neighborhood; and that was many years ago. Starving, terrified and full of fleas, it was quite obvious to us that a male had been cruel to him, because if my husband walked anywhere near him, he would shy away and make himself invisible. He was a small-statured brindle and white terrier-beagle mix (*terrorist*) with legs out of proportion to his long body and a tail that would curve over when he was strutting his stuff in front of any unsuspecting female in his vicinity. He would smile – literally – when he threw himself over on his back, begging for a belly rub, in seal-like fashion and then receive one. He lived for belly rubs. I would tell him that he had the best belly in the universe, and then he would smile some more. He'd literally throw himself down in front of you and take the risk of being trodden on for a belly rub. After his rough start in life, he took advantage of the copious amounts of food at Solace and became quite the little chubby chowhound, heralding the start of dinner with a most insistent bark that told us all he was happy and ready to eat, so could we please hurry it up. As his tummy filled out like a pumpkin, his back became flatter like a coffee table. Friends joked that he was our *pumpkin coffee table*, our *sausage boy*, even, on occasion, *Slim*. He had a whole host of nicknames.

When we rode horses in the vineyard, he was the best-behaved escort, staying out of the vines, away from the rabbits and yet close enough to be riding alongside you, unlike the other hooligans; but not so close you worried about him under hoof. As the years passed and he became less active, he was one of the 3 amigos who would do a lot of sleeping on the deck in their igloos, but not venture out much elsewhere, unless it was dinner time or an opportunity for a coveted belly rub. Baxter, Sophie and Roscoe – they were quite the threesome, all rescues and unlikely friends, but very mellow and secure in each other's company, tolerating the rest of the motley crew that would show up needing a bed for a night or two and a bowl of kibble. It was what we expected from them – you were rescued, and we took you in. You, in your turn, will accept the other rescues that come by; our unspoken rules of tolerance and acceptance.

After Baxter died, closely followed by Sophie, old *Smiley Boy* (another nickname), started to slow up quite a bit. He wasn't the cheery, perky chap we had enjoyed all these years. His breathing became labored. The seizures he had suffered with all his life became more frequent. In one day, he had 3 considerable ones that scared me. I realized, at the end of a long one, that he no longer recognized me. That was alarming. Though he continued to eat – our pumpkin boy – he was definitely less comfortable in his world. Then, one morning, he disappeared and was not barking excitedly for his morning cookie – most unusual. He was found circling and disoriented down below in llama land, where Sophie had also chosen to pass. It was time to let him rest. I'm never a fan of having to make that particular choice, but I do know that if they are suffering, it is past time. There is no more waiting for them to go naturally. At the vet, Roscoe went to sleep quickly, exhausted by the fabulous long life that he found at Solace with so many characters around him and the security of plenty of food and a warm bed to sleep in – not to mention the belly rubs and the love. He was quickly reunited with his two friends in the graveyard at Solace where, I'm sure, their spirits now play like the young things they used to be, where they run alongside the horses and feast on the yummiest bits of chicken and beef – some getting put in special hiding places for a rainy day. Like all good rescues, they never once lost their appetite for food, nor their fear that the supply would dry up.

On the day that Roscoe went to sleep, our Tucker gave blood at the local vets and saved another dog's life. And that is the circle of life and the right thing to do. Each sweet soul that passes takes a seat inside your heart with their quirky little mannerisms and their individual personas. You will never forget them. And, at the end of the day, you can rest peacefully knowing that you did the right thing by them from the day you met them to the day they were set free from their old bodies; and that is the best you can do. Though I miss my three amigos and all the others who went before, I know they loved their beautiful lives here at Solace and their spirits will always run free and easy on the breeze. We did our very best by them and they were so loved.

(2019)

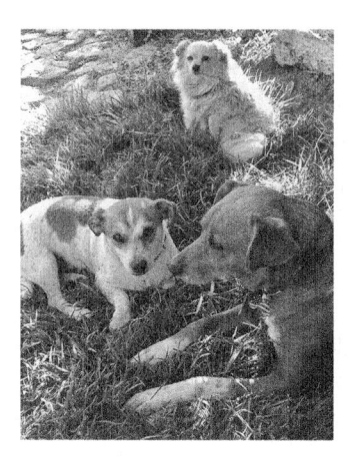

Plenty of room in rescue

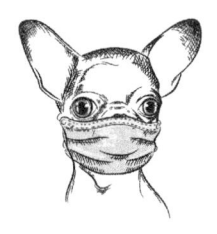

I was the co-founder of South County Animal Rescue (SCAR) back in January of 2016. At the time we were filling a large hole in animal rescue services in our area, and, since then, we have done many years of incredible work. Sadly, there is plenty of rescue work for everyone and the need only increases, as more kittens are born and more dogs are abandoned when they become ill or aged, or just difficult and untrained. There is also the wretched practice of backyard breeding that we come across all the time and that, though illegal, remains largely unpoliced.

I was asked recently about a new rescue that has opened up in our local area with a similar logo, but different name to ours. I wanted to clarify that this rescue is separate from SCAR. It was founded by some of the original SCAR volunteers, who have branched out on their own and are doing their own work. Again, sadly there is always more than enough rescue work out there for those brave folks who choose to walk in those shoes, and SCAR is happy to have the help out there in the field and aid the new group in their work.

This is not a race nor a competition. In the animal rescue world, all the groups need to help each other move towards the same goal – spaying and neutering as many dogs and cats as we can, educating the public about animal husbandry, and socializing and homing as many dogs and cats as possible, when they are abandoned and unloved. In short, we are all working to save animal lives. Social media is a great medium for this. Sometimes I feel overwhelmed by the amount of loving creatures smiling into the camera from Saint Elsewhere and hoping that someone will take a chance on them. Oftentimes, the shelters are crying out for help, especially from the rescue groups, to find a foster home for an animal and save its life. We all know that they cannot indefinitely have an animal in their care with no interest shown in them. Unless they can find a transfer out to another rescue or a home to place in while their forever home is found, the result is something I don't care to think about. It hurts my heart.

Early on in my rescue days, I was foster Mom to 11 dogs. I think some were actually mine at the time, but then my foster pup Mollie gave birth to 11 puppies, and it became complete pandemonium at my place. Fortunately, a good friend, who was also going to adopt Mollie once the puppies were weaned, took in the whole clan and successfully homed all the babies for us. That was one of the better rescue success stories that likely saved my sanity at the time.

These days I have 7 doggies of my own and I hadn't contemplated being a foster Mother again, since my hands are usually quite full. However, this old chap on Facebook caught my attention. A local rescue was pleading for someone to take a chance on him. He was so sweet he deserved a 2nd chance, but that didn't seem to be happening and the clock was ticking. Cooper, or Rufus as we call him, was a big old Shepherd with the most expressive eyes and such a sad demeanor. I reached out to one of the intake coordinators at SCAR and asked her if they could pull him and give him another chance at a happy life. Initially a foster was found, but then lost – and it was then that Solace needed to step up and be the safe harbor for another creature in need, just as we had done many a time before. Poor old Cooper had several medical issues that were being treated, but he still sported the sweetest disposition. He just wanted to be with his humans – even his temporary ones – and close by the other dogs. He settled in quicker than I have about ever seen. Cooper soon started finding his legs – likely he had been chained up much of his life – and trying to understand what a treat or a ball might be and why the other dogs loved them so much. He loves going for car rides and likes to watch the cars behind through the back window. Though he is a large dog and getting stronger all the time, his loving nature shines through. I have already learned a lot from being his Foster Mom.

I hope that he will find his forever home and not round out a pack of 8 at my place, but I'm okay if that turns out to be the case, because we will have saved his life and added another name and legacy to our rescue ranch, we call Solace.

SCAR and all the other rescues do fantastic and difficult work every day. They are mostly forced to fundraise in order for their rescues to function and they consist of teams of volunteers that spend most of their free time doing this amazing job. I take off my hat to all the groups whose goals are, ultimately, to save the lives of the innocent.

If you would like to support the group I founded, feel free to mail your donation to SCAR, PO Box 491, Soledad, CA 93960. Fundraisers are always happening and these are fun times for all with great food, live music, wine, often book signings by yours truly and silent auctions.

Thank you so much for listening to my animal rescue banter. Should you be interested in becoming a foster parent, there is an application waiting for you at scar.pet. Check out their posts on social media also – there are many darling creatures crying out for love and another chance at a better life. Maybe you could step up in one way or another, or you know someone that needs an adorable fur ball in their life.

One thing I have learned about animal rescue is that the work is never done. There are always more animals than we can rescue and more need than we can ever fill. Thanks to all the Animal Champions out there for all you do under some of the most difficult circumstances on this planet. There's a special place out there for you.

PS Cooper was adopted to Solace and officially became Rufus. To date he is the most beloved dog who lives out his days on soft beds and with the best food and cuddles.

(2023)

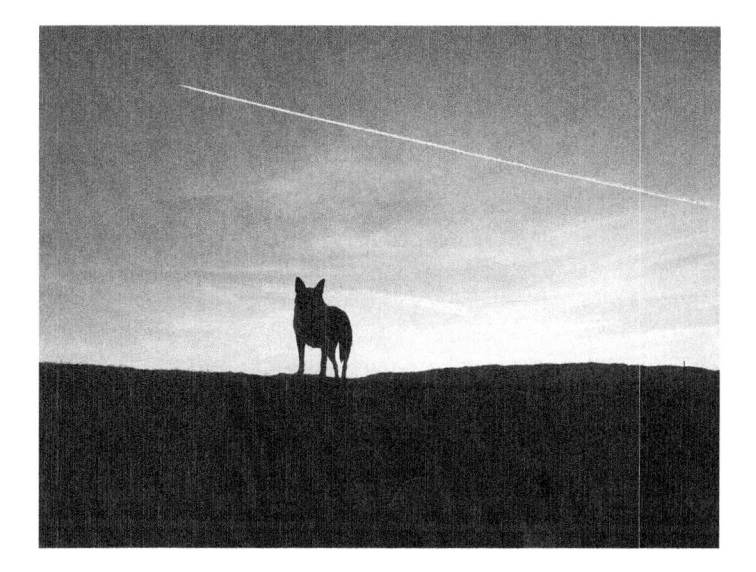

Sally Comes Home

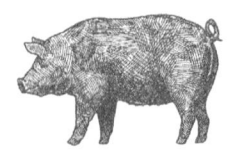

It has been a long time since we had a pig in the family. You read that correctly. Back in 2011, when my daughter was young, she raised an award-winning pig for the Salinas Valley Fair through the High School 4H. For rookies such as us, we did amazingly well; except that winning did not mean that Sally got to come with us that day. We mourned her for quite a time; not to mention the fact that not even a strip of bacon made it through our doors for months. We still talk about her with fondness; she taught us so much.

Over the years, I have casually glanced at ads for pot belly pigs – watched them joyously romping in people's family rooms. I do love a pig! Before Sally, I had no idea just how smart and fun they were; very intuitive indeed. Sally 1 would chat to us, play with the dogs, get super excited when she knew the marshmallows and strawberries were coming her way … she was a delight and we had raised us from a piglet when she left us at an award-winning 330lbs. Needless to say, that was our first and last foray into raising a market hog. None of us could stomach it again.

And then I noticed a slow-moving, black creature over at a neighbor's ranch. She was snuffling around in the dirt. "Sally!" I called out, randomly. "Sally O'Malley!" The dogs looked at me with disdain, thought bubbles hovering over their heads… "Oh no, she hasn't gone and rescued another dog, has she?" The neighbor seems to have animals coming and going; they never stay very long. I asked my other neighbor about the pig. He had been down there feeding horses. "If he wants to sell the pig," I broached cautiously. "I'll take her." And there it was. I had actually made a step forward or backwards, depending on how you look at it, into the swine world. "How much would you pay for her?" he asks me. (I'm thinking, whatever it takes.) '$100' Sold. Sally 2 was going to be mine. Soon a large black squealing creature was being delivered from the back of a pick-up truck to Solace in the arms of a very strong man. Fortunately, we had never dismantled the *Pygmy Goat Palace* from when Elvis and Charlie were young and needed to be contained. We would need to acclimatize Sally for a while. She screamed and cried. I felt so badly for her. I rushed inside and chopped up some lettuce, apples, carrots, banana … I even tried a marshmallow. She fell on the lettuce like a long-lost friend and chomped happily, almost humming with delight. I sat down and looked at her carefully. Initially I had thought she was young and pregnant; but now I could see she had been a breeding sow in her previous life. Now she was old and worn out; hence the $100 price tag. "It's okay Sally" I told her. "You can rest now. You are at Solace."

My daughter came flying outside. "Sally's home, Sally's home!" My husband was equally delighted. "O'Malley!" It had been 11 years since Sally left. It felt so good to have her back again. Then Max, our llama, caught sight of her and started screaming. Ever heard a llama scream? It's not pretty. Our llamas were terrified of this large black thing that could move about as fast as a tortoise. Sally didn't seem fazed though and was so appreciative of the regular food that was delivered and the fresh-water buckets to tip over and make mud pies out of. I take her breakfast in the morning and lay down in the straw next to her head. I love the smell and sound of a pig. I could get my head close to hers; but she screamed if I touched her, even very gently. I could not believe that humans had done a number on her when she had been nothing but a money-making machine for them. Even just a soft touch connection with a human terrified her. "It's okay, Sally," I told her. "We have all the time in the world for you to learn how to love a cuddle."

So now the Pygmy Palace has become the Piggie Palace and Sally has arrived at her forever home. It makes me miss my Winston White Horse all over again. He would have delighted at another friend to nuzzle and snort at. He would have loved the companionship of hearing her eat and watching her bask in the mud right next to his own palace of a stable. He certainly would not have screamed like a llama! Win had no issue with other creatures that had no equine resemblance. He loved the cats that visited with him in his stable and the goats that kept warm under his belly.

My neighbor tells me that the wanna-be rancher across the street, Sally's original home, now looked like he needed homes for his horses. "He seldom comes around to feed them," he tells me. The neighbor took over flakes of hay, since the horses had little grazing land left. "Oh no", I think to just myself; he has a Winston-looking horse. Enough time has passed that I am a likely sucker for a Winston-lookalike that needs a loving home. "Should we rescue the Winston?" I gently broached to husband, used to my raising a subject of such an ilk. (Normally a prelude to my next rescue.) "No", he says, categorically, not even looking up to catch my eye.

"We'd better give him a final chance!" I told the neighbor. "Let the landowner know that his tenant isn't taking care of his animals … maybe he will issue him an ultimatum."

And so, we watch, and we wait, and we deliver food. Neither one of us can bear to see a hungry animal. In the meantime, Sally's former abode is just a vague memory for her; of that I'm sure. She greets me with a bit of a whoop and a chortle these days, when I deliver her breakfast. She likes to eat her piggie grain first and then have the fruits and veggies for dessert. She lets me touch her and give her a back scratch. I love her; I just love her. My heart is so full. After 10 years away, Sally is finally back home.

(2021)

Sally meets Sibyl

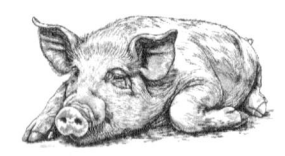

I was really happy at that farm. They gave me lots of food and water and mud! Oh, I love mud! They gave me straw to sleep on and room for my babies to snuggle. Whizz, the dog, would zoom into my stall and run around and around in the straw. She was so funny! Sometimes she would eat my grain, but I didn't mind. She was such a silly, scruffy little thing and there was always plenty to go around.

Then, one day, my babies left the stable and, all of a sudden, it was very quiet. Whizz came to see me, and she was very quiet. It was a spooky quiet. She cuddled up to me as if she was ill, but I knew she wasn't. Something was changing at the farm.

A man took me in a large trailer, and I wanted the Whizz to go with me, but she was not invited. Soon I was alone in a large pasture. It was full of dark and silence.

"Well?' A squeaky voice came out of the dark.

"Well, what?" I replied, looking around for something to eat in this strange place.

"Well, why are you here?" the voice said in the dark.

"I have no clue," I replied. "Where can a hungry pig get a meal around here?"

A large yellow, scrawny chicken stepped out of the shadows and pecked at the ground. "Better eat dirt, pig," she said. "He doesn't give us much to eat if ever. Lucky we like bugs!"

Sally looked around at the broken old shacks on the mini ranch and wondered why she would be left in such a place. This was terrible. No warm stable, no piglets to snuggle and no grain? She was very sad.

"Cheer up, chicken!" said the chicken. "I'm happy to share my bugs with you." Sally looked down dubiously at the black beetles in the dirt. "I really prefer grain, though my favorite is lettuce."

The chicken started cackling with laughter. "Lettuce, ha ha! Lettuce! What do you think this is – a salad bar?"

Sally lay down in the warm dirt and thought to herself, "Well this could be worse. At least I have a laughing chicken for a companion. Maybe I could learn to eat bugs."

A few days past and Sally never saw the grain she loved, or anything much. She nibbled on some of the horse's hay and tried some of the black bugs. She was not happy. Not happy at all. Finally, she was hauled into the back of a pick-up truck and then deposited into another field. "What on earth?" Sally thought and then her mind moved to grain and lettuce. Maybe, this ranch would give her some fruits and veggies.

"Morning Sal!" The lady moved down into the pen that Sally had made for herself, delivering not only lettuce, but yummy tomatoes, apples, bananas AND grain. She could not believe that she had got herself her very own salad bar. She was a little afraid of the lady after all these house changes she had endured in the last several days, but this was a good start. She crunched on the lettuce joyfully, sucked on the apples and licked the bananas.

"I like lettuce," said the yellow chicken. "Oh no, I don't share my lettuce," said Sally. "That is rare and divine food!"

"Fine, suit yourself," said the yellow chicken. "I was just coming over to introduce myself."

"Wait, wait," said Sally. "Here, have some of my lettuce! What's your name?"

"My name is Sibyl," said Sibyl, the yellow chicken. "I live here with my 4 sisters – Pauline, Maureen, June and Betty." "Oh. Lucky you! "said Sally. "I had to leave my 6 babies and come here."

"Awww, you must be lonely," said Sibyl. "Let's be friends. You give me a little peck of lettuce and my sisters and I will come and visit you often."

"Deal," said Sally and, all of a sudden, she felt very happy in her new pen with her lettuce and her apples and bananas and new friends.

(2021)

Saying bye to my boy

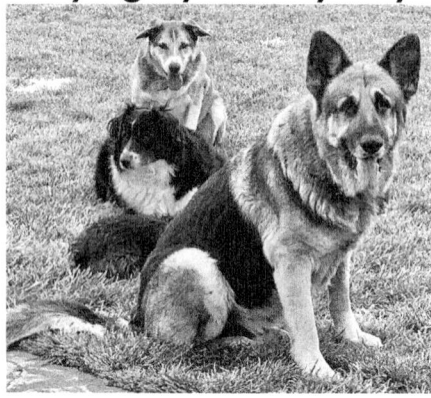

I couldn't take my eyes off him. He would stand up and then sit down. He wasn't comfortable. What to do, what to do? I couldn't move away from my standing position by the window of the house where I could see him up on the hill with the bright blue skies overhead. To my certain knowledge, he had only taken a sip of water in the past 24 hours. Likely 2 days since he ate anything, though I would still take him daily orchard hay to wherever he was hanging in the hope that he'd rally and show me his punchy personality from before. He had only nibbled a little the past few days. He was skinny and a shadow of his former formidable self. All the 8 years or so he'd lived with us, he was a huge purveyor of character. He had been unwell before and rallied abruptly. No, he wasn't interested in rallying anymore. He was shutting down and getting ready for his journey. The vet's shots had given him a little lift, bought him a few days perhaps, but now he was on the downward spiral and there was nothing more to be done; I could see that, though I could see little else. I sat down on the hill with him in the sun, petting his face, his neck, any part of him he'd let me. I sang Winston's songs to him that he seemed to like. His big brown eyes and long lashes fixed on mine. He seemed to be almost smiling. Such an unusually tame and gentle boy. His shearer would call him *maladjusted* because he was so tame. "He could hurt you badly," she insisted, "if he lets you pet him like a 400lb dog." I knew he wouldn't though – he loved people and especially me.

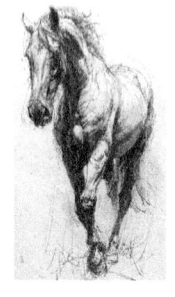

He had been sitting away from his brothers and the pesky pygmy the last few days, as llamas do when they are feeling unwell; but this morning the clan were all sitting close by – calm and comforting – not grazing or moving around, but just present at the impending passing of their brother in near ceremonial fashion. The dogs sat around us too, not bouncing up and down and competing for my attention, but just calmly waiting in the circular pattern of life and death we have come to know so well at Solace. This is my least favorite part of animal rescue and animal love – knowing when you have to let them go; knowing that you have done everything you know how to do, but it's not your plan to make or your decision to follow. I hate that part and I'm not good at it.

I went back to my position by the window in the house. I was supposed to be working on taxes and yet I was accomplishing nothing. If I couldn't see him, I couldn't stand it. Mostly his long neck was perched up on the hill, a little tired now, a little dipping down towards the ground. Then, all of a sudden, he stood up dramatically and I saw him fall over. I raced out the door, telling husband Demo was on his way. I'm not sure how I managed to race up and down the hills so fast, but I did. He was on the ground, when I got to him, breathing heavily. I nursed his head in my arms and sang Winston's favorite songs to him all over again. I bathed him in my salty tears and told him he would always be Chief Llama and I was so proud I got to be his Mum and to know his humor and his character for such a lovely long time. The other animals were all around us still. I told him it was okay to leave now; his spirit would always be with us at Solace. I told him to send all my love to Winston, Charlie, Buddy, Sophie, Roscoe, Joe and all the other characters in the kingdom where he was headed; the place where they don't age or hurt, and their beautiful spirits are free of their used-up bodies. We think it might be just a few feet above the land at Solace. He was calm and accepting. As he slipped away, a circle of eagles did a respectful dance overhead and his fellow animals sat in somber guardian stance.

Husband took him away to be cremated, so that he could always live inside the house with his friend Winston and enter the boundaries that had always fascinated him from his peering position through the glass sliding door on the deck. We would miss him horribly, but we will be always comforted by our amazing memories, plus glorious photos that were taken of him during his fabulous life on the ranch. He was a very special chap; irreplaceable, in fact. He will always claim a huge slice of my heart and I will never forget him.

Thankfully we were leaving to see our granddaughter a few days later and there is nothing like the vivacious, demanding spirit of a 5-year-old to remind you of the circle of life and the inevitability that, with new life, must come passings of older life. There is no room on the planet for all of us to stay forever.

(2020)

Harold Malcolm Democracy "Demo" died peacefully on President's Day, just like the King Llama he always claimed to be. He will be much mourned and missed. Solace was a very quiet and respectful place this week.

(2020)

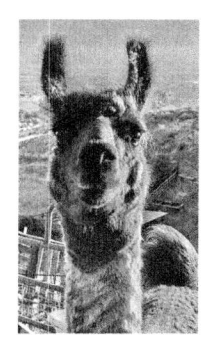

Small but beautiful things

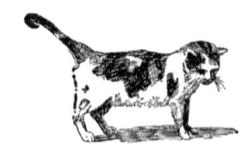

It was a long time ago. I had just moved into my office downtown and it was infested with mice. Though I loved the classic lines of my building – less the lack of heating and cooling – the hardwood floors and the character and flavor of a historic downtown base, I was less of a fan of the sprinting rodents I would catch out of the corner of my eye as I was trying to work. Oh, and don't even think about having any snacks in your desk drawers. Oh no, the most terminator-proofed plastic was just a wee challenge to my athletic rodents. Soon I realized that there was quite the colony of feral cats behind the building. The proximity of local restaurants probably perpetuated the growth of the cattery back there; but that's where the wiles of nature come into play. Cats and mice together equal, ultimately, less mice – it's just the law of the universe.

A spry calico kept coming to feed behind my office. I can never see a creature hungry, so I always feed strays, but I knew better than to leave her at the will of the natural world. She produced one litter off my watch. I homed the babies and then got Mama, as I called her, spayed. She was still pretty hissy and spitty in those days, but was a regular I could call over for tea and, within a split second, I would see her padding across the parking lot. In time, Mama would allow a short cuddle. I would pick her up gently, hold her close and, for no good reason, raise my eyes to the heavens and thank unknown powers that this whimsical calico trusted me enough to let me love on her a little. A few seconds of love was enough for her; but I felt humbled in her presence every time she allowed the connection. Even now, several years down the road, I still love to watch her sashay across the parking lot towards her dinner and me.

Calicos are a special breed. Well, truthfully, they are not so much a breed, as a mottled color mixture of a kitty that has somehow created, in my experience, a playful, smart and naughty, mostly female cat. Calico cats are predominantly female because their coloring is related to the 'X' chromosome, apparently, and two 'X' chromosomes are needed for a cat to have that distinctive tri-color coat. If a cat has an 'XX' pair, she will be female. Don't quote me on this; but this is what I understand, and, in all my years of rescuing calico cats, I have never encountered a male calico. A standard calico usually has a white coat with orange and black spots or splashes. The 'dilute' calico has the white coat, but also blemishes of smoky gray and sometimes a strawberry-blonde hue. The 'calibby' is the mix of calico and tabby, where the calico orange and black is often mixed with tabby stripes and this mix can bring a whole other level of naughty to the home! And these calicos often seem to cross my path.

My daughter had a beloved calico called Molly. She lived with her in her first apartment. Molly was an indoor cat and would occupy herself quite happily while my daughter was away at school or work, by carrying things up and down the stairs she thought were not positioned quite correctly. She had an enormous personality and would lay in wait for my daughter when she came home from work and, apparently, attack her with complete glee. When she calmed down, she was also super loving. My girl was her girl and that was all she needed. That also seems to be an enduring theme of the calico cat. They are completely, fiercely, devoted; but only to one person.

I rescued a Mama calico from a storm drain in Hollister. I didn't actually go into the drain myself – god forbid – but my friend did. She got all the kittens out and homed them, but no one wanted the mama. 'Will you take her, please?' she begged. Well, a calico, of course! Gotta love the challenge they bestow upon a human. I brought her home and she was a pretty wispy character; skittish and a bit feral. She decided that my mother-in-law, who was living with us at the time, was her human. Even though I had rescued her and given her a fabulous new life, I was pond scum to her, worthy of only an emphatic hiss or two. The senior in our household was her human and that was that. When the senior moved up north to Oregon, it was only fitting that the hissy calico would move with her. I can only imagine the fisticuffs that would have ensued had she been forced to stay with me – her rescuer, but never her human.

That's why I always giggle, when people tell me they have *rescued* a calico cat, because they are so fiercely opinionated and such incredible survivors, that they would never consider themselves to be rescue material. They would just deign to allow a human to spend time in their space, like an Egyptian princess, all poised and elegant in their calico glory.

"Mama!" I call for her in my sweet calico voice. "Mama, dinner time!" And soon she will casually stroll towards me, no hurry; her wet food can wait. Sometimes she allows me my special snuggle; other times, she turns her back on me and just wants her food and no bother. I love her for that. I am safe in the knowledge that she loves me and trusts that I will always come through for her.

My father tells me a friend of his has recently adopted an older cat. He sends me a picture. "Oh, that's a calico!" I comment, like a pro. "Oh ?" he responds. (We were always dog, never cat, people). I tell him a little about my adventures in life with the calico and he chortles. "Oh, Peter Marshall will have a wonderful time with him!" (His friend is always Peter Marshall, never just Peter!) "Her," I corrected him. "Her! They are almost always female." And then he tells me that I need to write a story to share my limited knowledge about calicos with the world and to remind people that, if they are lucky enough to be able to adopt or rescue one from a storm drain; not to let it hurt their feelings, if ultimately, they are not their human. Calicos are quite something to behold. If you like a challenge in life, a calico is for you.

(2021)

The Annual English Tea Party

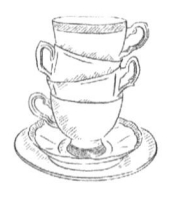

It has been a very long time since our last tea party. 2019, if I'm not mistaken. Prior to covid, the annual tea parties were very popular. Then covid came along and sucked all the fun, drove our traditions into the ground. Somehow it has taken us all a while to think about resurrecting the events we loved so dearly. Who dresses up and learns how to drink proper English tea out of proper English china? But why not? The people loved it, I enjoyed making English tea for everyone, folk actually paid to come to the event, and we even made some money for local charities! Is there a better way to spend a couple of hours on a Saturday afternoon? I think not.

The tea party concept was born back when Deborah was the reporter for the local newspapers and the Soledad Bee had their office next to mine. Deborah was very partial to a cup of English tea – with milk and sugar – and, most days, would race into my office and collapse in a chair. That would be my cue to put the proverbial kettle on and make a brew. She loved a decent cup of Yorkshire tea. It was normally easier to make a pot because one cup was never enough for Deborah. I would cover the china tea pot with a hand knitted *tea cosy* (like a coat for your pot) so that we could chin wag about the world and right things a little bit, whilst still keeping the tea hot. There is a little china teaspoon holder in my office that reads *Where there's tea there's life* and a lot of English people would agree with that. Having a bad day? Here's a cup of tea. Someone died? Have a cup of tea. Baby is born? Tea … you get the idea! My friend Sheryl too would love to share a cup of tea and a natter at the office back then and then she introduced her grandson to the tea-sharing concept, and they would enjoy little tea parties together. I like to think I have bought a little bit of England to these tiny farm towns.

So, the annual tea party grew and evolved from tiny little tea parties all over the valley. I realized how much people enjoyed the tea party – even if it was mostly just a conversation between two people over a hot cuppa – and thereby the concept moved into the bigger leagues. The Soledad Museum seemed like a great location to hold a neighborhood tea party and we decided to host it there as a benefit for the museum and the animal rescue together — maybe not two charities you'd put in the same room, but why not. Small towns have to work together for the common good.

Local friends got right behind the idea and started looking for china teacups and saucers in antique and charity shops. The ticket price would include the choice of china teacup and saucer to take home. It's amazing what lovely finds there are out there. Nobody buys china teacups anymore, it seems, so there are many to be found. My friend Paula Sarmento used to have quite the collection of them in her home on River Road, but I think they were more to feast your eyes on than to use. We did have some lovely tea parties at her home with her husband Bud and normally the much-coveted macaroons from the local bakery.

The tea party fundraiser was developing into quite the event. We would have local people make baked goods to serve with the tea and young people to serve the teas and top up people's cups. We would also have silent auction baskets and gifts so that people could give up just a little bit more money than they would otherwise for the token entrance fee. The youth cross country teams came to help out and they also learned how to serve and drink tea and got to take china cups and saucers home with them.

So, you'll be delighted to hear our event is back and we will be gathering in our finest teatime outfits at the Soledad Museum to enjoy some hot English tea and baked goods, conversation and silent auctions. Entry includes your own choice of china cup and saucer to take home with you. I'm hoping our ladies of the valley will remember this event fondly and gather their glad rags together and come out to support two worthy local charities. It has been hard putting events back together after the emptiness of covid, but here we are. Teatime is back and she cannot wait to see all of you. For my part, I'm happy I shall be returning to the homeland prior to the event so that I can buy fresh Yorkshire tea and be well prepared for the masses. I've already donated several sets of china from my own collection, gathered up my extra electric kettles and tea pots (along with tea cozies), so I am nearly ready to be your pouring host on the day.

We've said it before, but it does take a village for local charities to be successful. SCAR does an incredible job of rescuing, homing, rehoming and transferring dogs and cats in our local areas, as well as ensuring that all animals that are homed are spayed or neutered with up to date shot records. They are all volunteers who spend much of their own time and money working for the animals, so we appreciate all your help. As their co-founder, I could not be prouder of the charity and how far they have come since their inception in January of 2016. The Soledad Museum is a fine jewel in the crown of this valley and well worth a visit. While you sip your tea, you will be encouraged to peruse the exhibits and feast your eyes on the forefathers and their accomplishments within this beautiful valley we call home.

I look forward to seeing you there and pouring a delicious cup of English tea for you.

(2023)

The dreams of a rescue pup

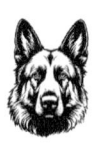

The beautiful dog awoke from its deep sleep dreamland. Before remembering his recent rescue, a bolt of concern ran through him from all those rude awakenings, and days and nights of fear. He could hear the comfortable long snooze of his new best friend just a few feet away. His tail slowly wagged once, and then once again as he took in his first morning sniff of his new day. He realized he was warm, and dry and had food in his stomach. And his old sad and fearful memories drifted back further as they had every morning since arriving, replaced with the joyful anticipation of a new day in his beautiful home, with his beautiful new family. His friend yawned widely. Rufus caught his eye, 'Is this doggie heaven?'

'No, but when we get there, there'll be a piece missing. This is it.

Eugene Ferris,
June 2023

Working in animal rescue is not for the faint of heart. Just when you feel as if you can take no more sad stories, welcome no more hungry and abused animals through your gate because your place is full, then along comes another and you cannot say no. The weight on your heart would be too much to bear, knowing the inevitability of the unwanted under these difficult circumstances.

We took in 3 cows, not knowing cows at all – or wanting to – (truthfully it was 2 cows, but Mama was pregnant, so yeah – 3). We have a fully grown boy steer who loves to govern the meadow and give us an understanding of why steers quickly become part of the food chain, but he's our pet, albeit a very large boy-cow with brute horns to match. We raised him from a youngster, and we struggle against doing what normal people might in this situation.

When my 3 amigos, my golden oldies – Baxter, Roscoe and Sophie – all passed in rapid succession to one another, Solace went down to a rather manageable level of 5 canines – a far cry from the 11 during the height of early-crazy rescue days. Oh, this is so doable, I recall almost congratulating myself. But then Stella arrived on our doorstep in a bird cage, Lizzie took my heart on the corner of Metz and 146 and Rufus, well, Rufus was going to be euthanized for lack of space at the shelter, and who needs that on their conscience, so he came along too.

'Can someone please go pick up that dog?' 'Will somebody please save that baby from death, he's out of time?' The cries are constantly out there for someone else to get out there and do the right thing for a creature in the animal world. Leaves a sour taste in the mouth. 'I cannot take him in,' comes another screech. 'I have a dog already!'

I do feel privileged to live where we do with some space around us. I try not to judge the well-meaning out there, who share and share and do nothing proactive to save the animals; but I like to think that Solace steps up where she can and helps wherever possible, even if it's not remotely convenient. It's what we do.

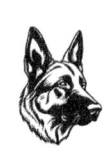

We took in Rufus – my first Shepherd – and he blended so quickly into the pack, it was as if he had just arrived like the Mary Poppins of dogs into a welcome situation that was expecting him all along. Normally, they say that a shelter/rescue dog coming from a nasty abandonment situation of being dumped and left to starve out in the wilderness will take a long time to acclimatize, settle, adjust, relax in a regular home. Not Rufus. He blended the first day he met everyone at Solace, as if to say 'oh, thanks very much for all the trouble. I'm home now. I knew I'd get there in the end!' Though there was a little adoption interest in him once we started posting him on social media, as an older boy with health issues we felt it better for him to just stay where he obviously wanted to be, amongst the family who had been waiting for him all along. Even now, a very short period of time since he arrived at Solace, I find myself questioning any little character quirks, as if he should have got over that by now. Err, slow down, tiger. It has been almost no time at all in the rescue scheme of things. And so, we make this rescue lark look easy, which it is not at all; but I have an expectation from my rescue pack that they accept rescues into their fold the way they were equally rescued. Mostly this works out.

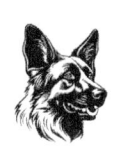

And then another shepherd desperately needed out of the shelter. Yet another shepherd. If you wonder why I bang on about rescuing animals and not buying from a breeder, just look around you at all the shepherds, huskies, pit bulls and more that deserve love and life. You do not need to be breeding any more dogs or birthing any more puppies if you take a good, honest look at the overpopulated dog world out there. Making money out of this dire situation is obscene. These poor rescue coordinators at the shelters are begging rescuers from other states to help, crying out loud to their local rescue organizations to dig deep for a foster to step up and save a life. Stop the backyard breeding, for crying out loud.

'I hate to ask, but I'm going to,' she approached SCAR. 'Could Lucy take in the shepherd? We are out of options for him.' Another older shepherd failed by humans and ignored by other people who might be able to help him. Of course, Lucy is going to help. The Sanctuary at Solace is underway for exactly the souls who deserve another chance at a better life. He may be 7, but that is not old. He may have some skin issues, but that is not an unusual thing. He can decompress in the sanctuary and then likely graduate rather quickly to the interior of Solace like the rest of them. Who abandons an animal? How some people live with themselves I do not know.

And so, another older shepherd arrived at yet another place that he knew not, a place he hoped he could stay at for a while, eat a lot of good food and drink a lot of cold water. He also hoped he could catch up with some sleep on a nice cozy bed and not be afraid of what might find him of a night when he was unprotected, or during the day when he was seeking scraps of food and dirty field water. He dreamed that his forever home was right around the corner, a place where he might learn a little about love. He wasn't going to create a big old fuss – he just wanted to feel safe and secure with his people. We are hoping all of this for him –

Lucy, June 2023

PS South County Animal Rescue (SCAR) pulled both Rufus (Cooper) and Marty from the shelter in order to save both of their lives.

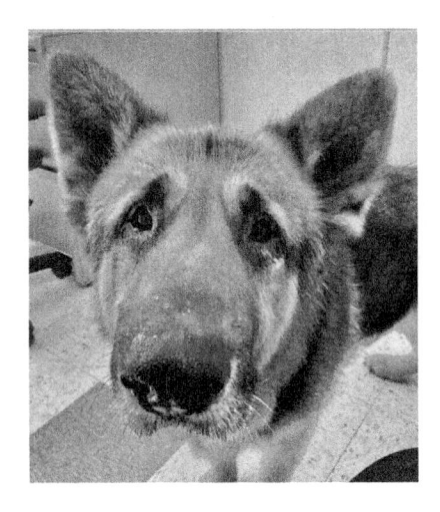

The Hen Palace

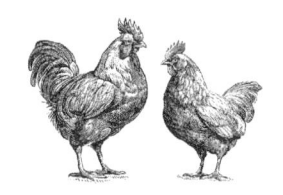

"I need to find homes for them," she said. "I have too many and they're stressing." Across the street, we have been building a chicken coop for well over a year now, so this wasn't a project that was going to get completed over the course of the weekend. But we did want chickens, we really did. We wanted the luxury of fresh eggs, once tasted never to go back to the store. Wait! We had an empty Kittingham Palace in Puppyland; could that work? All our spring cats and kittens had been homed. It could and would work. It might even spur the resident contractor onto finishing his coop sometime before Christmas. The plan was hatched, as it were. "What do I need to get started?" I asked my neighbor, the Chicken Lady. "Just some scratch and laying pellets … and some straw." I could do that. The first and last chickens I ever tended to were former battery hens – Queen Victoria, Henrietta and Charlotte. They lived out the end of their lives free-living and happy in our Secret Garden. I was very inexperienced; still am. But off I went, just a bit excited about the new critters that would be coming my way. I was off to buy scratch and pellets at the feed store like any normal chicken lady – like I knew what I was doing.

"Which ones do you want?" she asks me. (I'm at the chicken lady's house). "Well, I think it's going to be more like which ones can we catch!" I commented, as I watched the wings and feathers flapping around in the dust at all this disturbance of 3 humans in their pen. That was a comedic exercise if ever I saw one; but finally, we trapped 5 ladies of different shapes and colors in our dog crate. They were obviously going to be the perfect ones to move across the street to our place.

I was warned that the ladies might stress further for a few days in their new abode and not produce any eggs, so I shouldn't worry. I sat down on my small stool in the newly named *Chickingham Palace* with them and we had a little chat. "Now ladies," I tell them. "This is a really fabulous place to live, and I can promise you new and interesting things to eat, lots of doggie barking and a fair amount of human interaction. Let's start with some zucchini and some cucumbers. How about some snails? Rice? Oh rice …" And there I had them – even more than the snails. They loved the stuff. Well, this is easy, we always have bits and pieces of food left over. That night I was thrilled to see my first perfect egg. Within 3 days, I had scored 5 fresh eggs and how amazing they were. Creamy and deep yellow, so rich and splendid-tasting. How had I survived so long without my own hens? So now they have graduated to their own roosting perches, and we are starting to look as if we know what we are doing in this chicken business with our 5 perfect ladies totally a part of the family.

Meanwhile, next door in the Secret Garden, my 3 turtles must be wondering what on earth is going on with all that squawking and hollering; but it hasn't slowed their snail appetite at all. I find myself digging through the damp grasses and foliage in the morning looking for juicy, chunky snails. I talk to the baby snails: …"oh you're spared; you need to grow a bit. I'm going to take Mama if you don't mind." I'm thrilled when I find a big old batch and go sit on the side of the pond, calling the turtles over to come and have breakfast. They are a funny lot. This week I even caught the snails riding on the backs of the turtles, which presented a hilarious picture. And who said snails aren't smart! So, at Solace, we've had some fun and interesting things going on this week and we are very happy with the new additions to our family. I nearly adopted a baby goat just to shake things up, but someone got there before me … and I said I wasn't having any more goats in any case, so that was just as well. In the countryside you are surrounded by gifts – feeding and nurturing your critters is an important component of this delightful circle of life.

(2019)

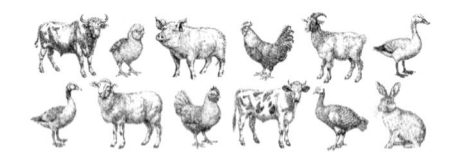

SECTION 3

Me & The World

Introduction to –
Me & The World

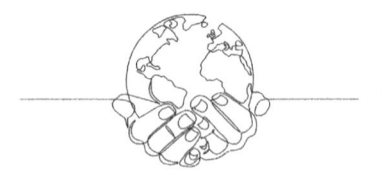

Oh, my word, this is a very eclectic collection of stories – from the King's Coronation in England to concerts in Nashville in high summer to my first adventure with Covid and the experiencing of lousy customer service one can come across these days – even in America, ahem.

This collection is all over the place in color and texture, highs and lows, but it also reminds me that it is important to get out into the world while you still want to, regardless of whether it gives you your first dose of covid in return. This is a recurring theme in *Tomorrow Is Not Promised*. It also reminds me of how primal our homing instincts are and how we travelers feel when we are finally home again.

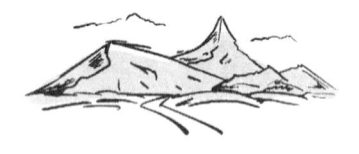

The world can be a cruel place, but also fabulous. Almost in the same breath. I have learned many things in the last 5 years and one of those things is to never take my homes in England or America for granted.

I hope you enjoy the wild ride prevalent in these tales.

Let me know if you do – or don't.

lucymasonjensen@gmail.com

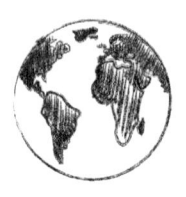

A rare and crazy adventure

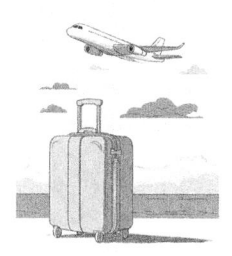

It all began in regular fashion. You are getting ready to go on a trip; so, therefore, things get really het up at work – not in a good way – and you are putting out fires, like California in summer – why does that always happen? Finally, you have put all to bed that you are able, and you are on the airbus to the international terminal, passport and important documents in hand. Check. That is the beginning of a good trip. (There have been times when I have missed the bus; not such a good start!) You are cruising along listening to your music and enjoying the first vistas of the San Fran skyline, remarking in your cheery head that there is so little traffic on this sunny day. This is when you receive a blocked call from the San Jose Police Department. Your world stops, though the bus keeps going. The driver had somehow left your case on the curbside at San Jose airport, and it could be now found nice and snug and safe at the Lost and Found. In San Jose Airport.

Funnily enough, I had remarked to the driver, when he was loading my bag, how curious it was that there were so many of the same bag in the hold – not just the same color, the same brand – you think he would have clocked that he needed to be just a little bit more careful. One would think. I got just a tad upset when I was informed about the fate of my bag, as we thundered northbound towards my airline with no bag in place. The driver told me he didn't feel safe with me sitting behind him, like I was going to clock him in the head or something as we whizzed along in the fast lane. At least he wasn't texting and driving at this point. The airbus company was not very helpful either. They told me that they couldn't really help me, except that they WOULD reimburse me for whichever service I found to collect my bag – or not. They couldn't have the next bus stop to pick up said lost bag, since they were not allowed to leave the bus unattended. I could not believe it. I was either going to fly without my luggage, or I was going to have to use modern technology at its best and have Uber pick up my bag. The first couple of calls with Uber scared the drivers so much they disconnected the calls. Finally, Fahim in his Porsche Carrera took me on. "Oh yeah I do luggage pickups all the time!" He had a smiley voice. I could have kissed him.

I ate a little lunch with a large glass of white wine and waited for Fahim. Soon-ish, lo and behold, there was my black and yellow beauty sitting sweetly and fairly untarnished like a smug bee on the tarmac of the International Terminal. $107 later and we were reunited, just in time to check said bag and cruise through security. You would have thought that the airbus service would be checking that somehow the bag and owner were safely reunited with one another? It was, after all, their driver's fault that he LEFT MY BAG ON THE SIDE OF THE ROAD! Nope. Customer service at its finest.

It was a lovely flight indeed after all that baloney. I had treated myself to a $124 upgrade and was very comfy, the plane being only about a quarter full. Arriving at Terminal 3 and cruising through passport control like a boss, or at least a British Citizen, I had some time to kill before my mandatory day 0-2 covid test at the airport. I enjoyed a nice flat white coffee (like a strong latte to you) and strolled with my lovely black and yellow bag in tow to Terminal 2. This is quite a long way in actuality, since Heathrow Airport is a gi-normous complex. All well and good until I see the line – or queue – for the covid testing. Nooooo! I scream inside my own head. Fortunately, there was someone checking the thousands of people who were clutching their vital paperwork in hand and wildly hoping they were in the right place. I wondered, briefly, how many folks would skip out on that little mandatory requirement and take a chance that the covid police would not have the energy or resources to be checking that everyone had followed the rules. You can have thoughts like that after 10 hours on a plane, an 8-hour time difference and unusual bag dramas. "Oh no," the nice cockney lady tells me in her fluorescent jacket. "YOUR testing place is OUTSIDE the airport!" Outside, like around the corner? "Oh no, you will have to get a cab." Hmmm. The instructions very clearly stated Terminal 2 and not outside the airport. My wish to follow the covid rules was quickly waning. I grabbed a London taxi and he proceeded to dump me in the middle of nowhere; a covid parking lot to be exact. I couldn't help but wonder how on earth I would find my way to London from here. Quickly tested in the covid parking lot (throat and nose, hate the throat part) and the parking lot director pointed me towards an alleyway, leading to a road, where I might be able to take a bus to take me back to the airport. At this point it was drizzling and my black and yellow bag was no longer feeling quite so light and fabulous.

I finally jumped on said bus where I proceeded to limp onto an underground tube station that would then take me downtown. Goodness me, what a palaver. Leicester Square was where my hotel was hiding, and I say hiding because I had to walk twice around the sizeable square to find it. I asked the nice doorman at the Radisson, and he told me they had available rooms at his place, but I had already paid for my hidden room, tempting though that was, especially since it was raining proper by now. He did steer me in the right direction though – more than I can say for the bus company – and soon I was in the dry. The first room the Victory Hotel tried to give me didn't have a window and I told them I couldn't sleep in a windowless room. It was upwards from there, however, and I soon got a back-alley room with an inoperable window. I had to be happy with that. I had arrived, I had my luggage with my clean clothes. I could take a shower and sleep a bit. What more can you ask for after that kind of adventure? Oh, you can ask for a lot apparently. I managed to squeeze in two West End plays in one day and a late night Greek meal. Yes, it was that kind of crazy adventure.

(2021)

Above all else

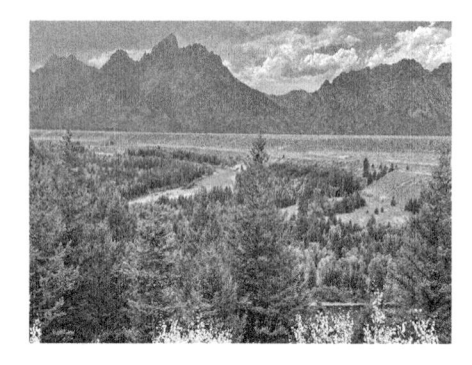

The definition of kindness is the quality of being friendly, generous and considerate, according to the Oxford Languages, wherever they might hang their hat off the Google imprint. The true meaning of being kind is doing intentional, voluntary acts of kindness. Not only when it's easy to be kind, but when it's not – at least that is my take on it.

In the past month and a bit, I have witnessed enormous acts of kindness – human compassion of the best kind; the sort that occurs when no one is looking or taking inventory of the good deeds on display. When my daughter and her boyfriend were slapped up and down and turned a few times over by life and the chariot she can ride in, not to mention their Ford Truck that was completely destroyed, I felt so sad and desperate for them. Not only was she injured, but the pair of them were also beaten down and depressed, having lost their dream vacation, their truck and most of their possessions – not to mention the health of my daughter's back and psyche. It was a brutal time. I did not know what I could do to cheer them up, especially my daughter who was unable to work and still is. She also seemed to be developing agoraphobia there for a while. Her boyfriend was forced to deal with not only her but also all the annoying adulting that ensues when you are required to manage insurance companies, adjusters, police … all because a wrong-way driver with dementia and no driving license was allowed to take the wheel of someone else's car and cause destruction and mayhem.

People came out of the woodwork and offered up kindness in her purest form, as soon as the word got out that there were some hard-working innocent young people that needed their help. They made us dinners, offered assistance, contributed to a *Go Fund Me* account and sent multitudes of kind words over the ether – not to mention visiting us in the hospital when we could really use a kind and familiar face, cupcakes and coffees. Complete strangers offered to help – not for any reason other than they wanted to. That completely blew my mind. In the past I have felt that some do good things when they think others are looking. But, in this type of situation, when a couple of kids are down on their luck and they happen to be our kids, you don't really expect such an outpouring of love and support from people that didn't even know them. "Glad to help!" one party noted. "Sending healing love to Aaron and Francoise,' another posted. "Wishing them all the best," chimed in another. Nobody was standing by taking the head count of those who wanted to help. And this got me thinking. What if we all performed random acts of kindness when no one is looking?

I love the downtown pantry and mini libraries you can see in our small towns. Help yourself, they call out to the world at large! Need that pack of rice or a couple of books for your kids? You just take what you need. Have extras yourself that you could easily part with? Just fill up those puppies. I love that they can sit on our streets and fill the needs of those who might not have quite enough, without being abused or vandalized. An automotive repair company downtown collects clothing for the needy. Not because it helps their automotive fixing sales, but because they believe it is the right thing to do; and it is. I have to believe that, when you do the right thing with unadulterated kindness in your heart, the rest will follow.

Almost a million years ago, I was new to this country and living on the Bayou in Louisiana. A very long way from my present home in California, I can tell you! We were residing in a trailer, which was great as a roof over the head, but it had no furniture and the floor in the bathroom showed the ground below. Lizards used to come and play in the trailer and rest on the walls. Sometimes they would fall off the walls and onto you. There were flying bugs, the like of which I have never seen before. I remember grabbing an outdoor hose at the trailer and seeing a water moccasin ricochet off the rubber. Everything was pretty hand to mouth at that time, but we didn't ask for help. That wasn't in my nature.

It was Thanksgiving Day and there was a knock at the trailer door. A lady tried to give us a basket full of yummy things so we could enjoy our own Thanksgiving. It was so very heartwarming and kind. We couldn't accept the gifts, the basket full to the brim with food treats and items we could never afford at the time. There were many more people way worse off than us, we thought. The lady seemed confused, as she backed away from the door with the basket still in her arms. She couldn't believe that an empty house with two people and a dog would not be accepting of a kind basket donation on Thanksgiving Day. I look back at that day and smile a little. I would likely never accept help like that if I have the means to work and help myself. But sometimes life puts you in a corner and it's okay to accept a little help. Especially when it's for young ones or animals.

The help that poured in for my daughter recently honestly helped her with her recovery – both mental and physical. From my dad with his fishing pole dollar replacement offerings, to old friends and the generosity of so many dear people that lifted her up when she felt beaten to pulp and offered her hope for a better day; gave her an open-armed chance to forgive the lady who hurt her and the opportunity to begin to heal from multitudes of injuries – some you could see and others you couldn't.

Oftentimes, it is not what happens to you in life that is key to a successful recovery, but how you respond to it. When you are aided by so many loving, giving hearts that wish you well, wish you better and wish you back, your return journey to a kinder life will be a lot smoother.

Thanks to all of you, pure and generous hearts, not to mention the power of modern medicine, Francoise and Aaron will ultimately be just fine. Their spirits are much better and their sanity intact. Francoise is healing well, and Aaron just managed to qualify for a replacement truck that he absolutely loves. I shall be sure to return all of the favors in due course.

Thank you, beautiful people. We love you all.

(2021)

Be grateful

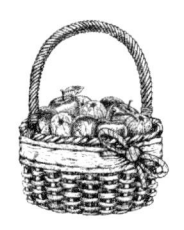

It is beyond time to show gratitude in our world. Though Thanksgiving is now just a belly-filled memory away and the shops are already over-filling with Christmas cheer, our gratefulness should extend beyond our own dining table and under our fancy tree-skirts to the world outside. 'Do something good when no one is looking,' said someone famous. We should do that all year long, but especially this time of year when it can be cold and wet outside and the loneliness inside is so very enhanced. I have food in my fridge, a warm house, companionship and an ability to work and buy more than just the essentials. I am so very fortunate. I also remember when I wasn't. It was my first year in the U.S. – 1988 – and we were living in a trailer on the Bayou outside Baton Rouge. Truthfully, a bit down on our luck. This story will be covered more fully at another time; but serve to say we had no furniture nor possessions except for a beat-up old rock & roll van. We slept on the floor of this old double wide next to the bayou and considered ourselves lucky at the time, especially from where we had come. Our neighbors put our names forward for the Salvation Army Thanksgiving baskets, donations to the poor. We were so humbled and overwhelmed; but we couldn't accept them. In our book, we had the ability to work, we had a fairly dry roof over us, and we just were not that poor. You never forget things like that.

Move stage forward about 30 years and I was working down in King City and needed a cup of hot tea that I could easily afford. I waited in line and noticed a skinny young man sitting in the corner with an empty cup. He looked so downtrodden and depressed. He left his grubby baseball hat on the seat and went to use the bathroom. "I'll be right back," he said to the cashier, lest somebody throw away his hat. It was quite obvious he had nowhere in particular to go, and the weather was frightful outside. I bought him the largest hot sandwich they served in the place and asked the cashier to give it to him when he came out. A simple act of kindness that I could easily manage. How many of us just walk on by in our own little cloud and don't pay attention to the basic needs of others. If you can do better, please do. I hope he felt a little less desperate after his sandwich.

There's a non-profit group down in King City called Sun Street Centers. They do good work all over our County. They are looking for gently used warm clothing, shoes, boots, jackets and so on for men and women. Decent clothes to wear? Is there anything much more basic than that? Most of us have our closets full to the brim with things we barely use. I'm going to dig out some of ours and get it to this group. It's a small thing, but why not. It's called humanity. Years ago, on that same Louisiana adventure, someone did the same thing for me so I could get a decent job.

In the spirit of the season, I was working on my *Thank You* page or *Acknowledgements*, as you can find in most published works. My e-book of *The Animals Teach Us Everything & Other Short Tails* has just come out on Amazon. I skipped through it and then realized that the very important *THANK YOU* page was missing from the finished work. I had seen it on a proof, and here it was darn well missing. Would people notice or care? They might well; since thanking folks is an important part of daily communications and someone would likely notice my lack of care and courtesy. And now the e-book was going to be morphed into the printed book and since it had taken me such a long time to get to this point, I was reluctant to try and make any further changes, since I might then receive the version 3 I had recently received as a proof, or something quite other. Gosh, communications are harsh – even, or especially, in this digital age! So I decided to leave the *Thank You* page out of it for now and just have a personal thank you card printed up like a photo and put it inside the printed book as a bookmark. It seemed like a reasonable compromise, especially since I wanted to actually have printed books in my hands to give away at Christmas or, laughing, accommodate the holiday rush. I did have to smile a bit knowingly, though, as I began my *Gratitude* column and swallowed rather painstakingly at the prospect of there being no thank you page in my book – that is rather going against the grain, but that's life, isn't it. Full of compromise!

"How's it coming along, Lu?" one of my loyal readers asked. "Ugh. So. Tired. Of. It!" I groaned in response. I know many a writer who struggles with what happens after you finish writing and this tome is at least a year late in publication date, so I'm rather seriously sick of it to be honest. But I will finish it, imperfect or not, and I will always smile at the missing *Thank you* page and the go-around I needed to make to get it off my dusty old desk and in front of my loyal readers.

During this season of thankfulness, try and pay attention to the skinny guy in the corner who needs a sandwich and be kind to the authors who make mistakes in their well-intended publications. Also, if you can find time to dig out some nice warm clothes, shoes, boots and jackets for the local Sun Street Center, that will help a lot of people during this inclement weather in the beautiful State we all call home. It's all good stuff and ensures that human beings are still better than robots or computers or publication mistakes.

(2021)

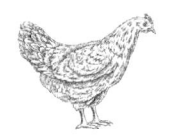

Busy people

Busy people stay busy. And not much alters with time, despite your best efforts to spend more time relaxing at home with a novel, or … ahem … working on your own novel.

As many of you know, I have been trying to work on my *Rosie* project. It's a very absorbing effort when I make the time to work on it, which seldom happens at home. Home is, simplistically, about animals, family, work. This year, I managed to royally mess up the renewal courses for my notary commission, so I have been scrambling to take care of that, when I could have cruised through it at the end of last year without a bright red emergency renewal letter in sight. And why didn't I do that? Because I was so busy doing other things. In my own defense, I was juggling a lot of things like a royally sick husband, but I still could have made it so much easier on myself. Now my commission will expire before I have the new one in place. I had to do a 6-hour class, instead of 3, and instead of cruising over to beautiful Monterey for my test, I must go to Modesto and take the exam there. Oh, and it will likely be a few weeks before I am all commissioned and bonded and able to do the work again. All my own fault.

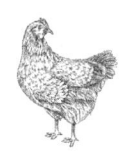

In this modern world, you can spend a lot of time doing inanely busy things like resetting passwords, trying to get a message to extricate a file or bypass privacy systems that make you howl with impatience. Recently I was so wound up in knots, I asked the lady to please just mail me the wretched document, since she said she was not allowed to email it and the privacy extrication wasn't working. Busy work accomplishing nothing.

"I'd like to order 10 copies of your 'Winston Comes Home' book", he said. Oh, how nice! Another person asked me for 2 copies. It was published in 2014, why the sudden interest? I hunted around in my book boxes. I had one dog-eared copy left. Hmm. Never thought that through, did I. I tried to contact the old publisher. They had gone out of business, sold to another company. Ok, that should be easy. Contacted the new company, no reply. Sent another message. Same response. Called. Same. I figured their lack of customer service must be because my book has died along with its old publisher. It is no more. What now? Let it die? No, that's a bit unthinkable. Re-do it? What, more busy work, when I'm trying to find the time to work on my Rosie book … plus get that blessed notary commission finished up?

I contacted the publishing service of my last book. Thank goodness they were still alive and would love to help me reconstruct my book. I remembered my sister Rosie telling me that there were elements of that book that could have been better, especially the photos. Well, look here, sister, we now have the opportunity to fix that. Looking back, I also wasn't a huge fan of the cover. Another superb possibility to improve the old beast. Amazingly enough in the kleptomaniacal depths of my computer files, I was able to find the e-proof from the book that I am hoping the publisher will be able to use and extract/change the items that need to be altered. I am also hoping that the whole project will be off my desk and onto his this coming week, so that I can revert my focus onto all my other busy priorities. Plus get back to my Rosie book. Anyone else have these 4 steps forward, 6 back frustrations in life?

Then I look at the calendar and it's time for my 2nd Moderna shot. The first put me in bed and gave me a few days when I got nothing accomplished. I cannot afford to have that happen this week. Make sure you eat and take Tylenol or Advil before the shot, the pharmacist tells me. Give yourself the best chance of having less side effects. We will just go along with that and hope that my days can line up in a more orderly fashion and allow me to complete more things. There is never enough time in the day, week, month. The plan was to have my Rosie book to the publisher by the autumn and here we are going back to a 2014 publication and recreating the wheel. Time will tell if my Rosie book will make it out to the public in time for the holiday buying season!

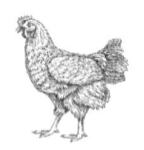

Oh, and I have my first book signing coming up, hosted by Scheid Vineyards. Because of the pandemic, *The Animals Teach Us Everything & Other Short Tails* never got the opportunity to receive the exposure I had hoped for. At the end of the day, I was quite pleased with the publication and a little sad it never got the lift-off I thought it deserved. So, there's another busy thing to fill up an afternoon, though I do so appreciate the opportunity to get back to *normal* life again!

Now, back to the uncertain week of my Moderna vaccine and my miserable notary commission efforts. Busy people need to be more organized in their busy lives and get their priorities straight and in line. Otherwise, you may end up with the kind of basket of mess I have created for myself. Just because I have 4 diaries does not mean I am the organized person I wish I were. Note to self; must do better next week.

PS The Moderna vaccine threw me into bed for the best part of 24 hours. Now I am behind again.

(2021)

Grandmas gone wild

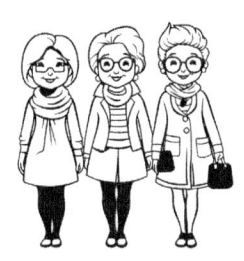

With the world starting to re-open, we were hoping to have a bit of a newsie reunion. Several of us from the newspaper industry had remained friends over the years, enabled by the easiness of social media and genuine friendships that survived the test of time and variation of lives and locations. After the dire lack of vacations in 2020, it was time to revisit some fond connections. A Vegas trip was planned to see one of my besties. She had relocated from Salinas a while back and it was time to catch up. Initially I had thought that there would be several on the *Newsie Girls Gone Wild* adventure in Sin City; but it whittled down gradually to a manageable party of 3; a triangle of ladies of a certain age we fondly called *The Grandmas*, because we are.

Staying at the new Circa property off Fremont Street set me off with a certain exhilaration, since it boasted no less than 6 swimming pools, not to mention a multi-sports screen the size of an airplane. How bad could that be? Though the room rates were certainly up there with the best of them, I love to be in the water wherever I go, so water it was.

Curiously enough, my Vegas friend is just finishing up her first book about *Common Courtesy*, which, sad to say, was a bit lacking in the new Circa hotel. The hotel guests should have been feeling lots of love from the largesse of their room rates, but this was not the case. No coffee pot in the room, no service of any kind actually (my friend never did get the fresh towels she requested from early in the morning until late at night.) Though hotels will certainly blame the corona virus for about anything these days, I think not cleaning a room should serve to provide a discount for the paying customer. Nobody asked, nobody checked. I was, understandably, upset to note that I ran out of toilet paper on my last day. If you are not going to service a room, you had better at least stock it for the duration of the stay. As a former hotelier, I know how the small stuff can really mount up to big chunks of displeasure over the course of a few days stay. And nowadays there are customer service hotspots like Trip Adviser to really get *The Displeased* going.

Circa does have lovely pools, no doubt about that, and the largest screen for sports you have ever seen. However, unless you pay a gazillion dollars, (no discount for the hotel guest), you will not be able to use anything except the scarcely populated chairs that are not right next to the water (with no shade cover on the chairs at the weekends). We had enquired about renting a cabana for the day and that was an obscene $4000. Not all the pools were open all the time, so guests were jammed into small spaces of water on too many occasions, which is not a great idea for the covid-phobic among us, let alone general policy that the masked police were fond of informing everyone located near the water; but never mind the super-spreaders actually inside the 3 feet of water. The cabana sheriffs wouldn't even let us put our towels on the chairs of an empty cabana because we hadn't paid to play. The scene didn't inspire huge feelings of love from the resort to the guests. They only seemed to care that you were spending more money than you had already. "Well, that's Vegas," you might say. But Vegas or no, you do have a tremendous choice when it comes to booking a hotel and they should be mindful of that once the novelty of their property wears off.

My friend had booked a special twilight cocktail hour in the Legacy Club at the hotel with panoramic views of the City and expensive cocktails to boot. The Foot Police had elected to bestow the difficult rule-enforcing task upon a very slight young hostess. She needed to tell the well-intentioned patrons of the Legacy Club that flip flops and tennis shoes were not to be worn on the upper decks. Oh, that poor chick. Since most people go to Vegas with only those items of footwear in their luggage, she was in for a long night. Fortunately, the manager cleared my expensive Sketchers for lift off and we were finally allowed out on the roof, though we did not get the benefit of the reservation we had made. We were, however, successful in stealing An Other's seating situation when they failed to appear. It seems as if you have 6 minutes to appear for a reservation in Vegas and then it evaporates. Sometimes, the reservation is not even a proper reservation. Apparently, only a suggestion?

Everything continues to be fast and furious in Las Vegas, *Corona* or no. Taking in the color of Fremont Street on a Friday night – few masks, let alone mask police in sight – I found it interesting that I no longer feel comfortable in a crowded situation. I do not want to be in spitting distance of anyone, let alone a mass of marauding folks that, perhaps, still believed covid was just a hoax. At my urging, we took off down the side streets and found ourselves in a rather magical city garden bar, complete with fairy lights and your own private see-saw, if you knew how to find the secret entrance in back. I found myself squealing with joy from delight as we bounced each other up and down on that old flashback from Childhood. Moving on, again off the beaten track where restaurants were touting a 90-minute wait, we discovered another gem for dinner – a classic old-style establishment, the kind that boasts signed photos of old crooners on the walls and dark wood paneling. I devoured what was likely the best pot roast, mashed potatoes and gravy to ever cross my path. It also exhibited lovely customer service, quite the antidote to our poor customer service impressions previously. The following night, we devoured possibly the best Italian food I have ever enjoyed, again off the Strip.

If you are headed to Sin City for some fun in the sun, make sure you do research before you go. Newest does not mean best. Check out the reviews on *Trip Adviser*, where I shall be positioning my review, right after I have contacted the Management at the resort; not to complain, but to give them the opportunity to do better. When we know better, we do better? *Grandmas Gone Wild* had a super time catching up in this wild of wildest cities. And now it's back to work and to a relatively more peaceful world of fixing a broken septic and paying bills.

(2021)

Hope is springing forth

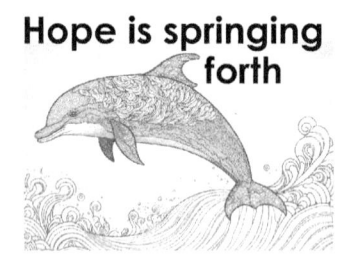

'Tis the time of the dippy doves and dizzy flutter-byes, the swaying orange poppies and white tree blossom. 'Tis the time for the green-green sprouts of hope to anchor themselves way down in the rich soils of our homes, time for the tipsy butterflies and the whooshing dragonflies, drunk on the wind, to show up at our windows and doors. The turtles are up on the banks of the pond once more, basking in the sun, their rich green shells rejuvenated after their winter sleep and their tummies hungry for the fresh snails plucked from stealth-crawling up and down the fruit trees. The birds of the world have showed up, calling out their shrill voices high in celebration of the new spring, new life, new hope. They are nesting and giving birth to their young, pecking tiny bugs from the house and splashing in the fountains. Over in the meadow, the green and fuchsia-flush hummingbird guards the nest and swoops at anyone or thing near the bush. And then she's off again, way high up into the ether blues, playing on the wind and decelerating as she comes in for landing once more. She let me photograph her on the anniversary of Winston's death. I sang to her, as you do, and decided she was one of his spirit creatures, checking in to let me know that my beloved's enormous spirit lives on in the meadows of Solace; as if there were any doubt. Our starlings have returned, as have our bluebirds, magpies, meadowlarks and more. Generations of birds return to nest at our place; we always leave the nests intact, so they don't have to work so hard every time they return from who knows where. Strutting grey collar doves strut and posture in antiquated courtship mode and coo in a way that shakes my memory box of youth.

I have taken to stroking my trees, (often in pursuit of afore-mentioned snails for my lady hens and turtles). I talk to them and water them, stroking the wise old trunks that give you a grounding sense of time and place. They give so much and expect so little; they are my old friends and are to be cherished. My ladies in Chickingham Palace bestow so much joy. The sight of them thundering towards the gate on their chicken run and scrabbling after whatever taste-treats I might have for them that particular time makes me hoot with laughter. I clean their stable and make damp areas around so they can scratch for bugs – they are safe and loved. They bask in the morning sun and vocally herald the arrival of new freshly laid eggs that delight us so. The more I cook for them and feed love into their little bodies, I do believe, the more they trust me.

It's time to pull the weeds up and think about the garden and the yard. It's time to wash off the cobwebs and consider maybe a fresh coat of paint on the shelter that protects you and yours. Make time to enjoy the longer days, the crushing sunsets, the starry skies. Awake in the morning to the promise of a better day, a chance to do fabulous, or even just simple, things all over again. Be grateful for your ability to see, to smell, to hear. Don't take for granted the fact you can walk unaided and breathe the airs. You are able to move your body, feel your heartbeat and swallow without assistance.

So many things we take for granted, until things are taken away. Then we question and we fear the unknown world outside our door. We miss our perceived freedoms, but we still have so many to enjoy and others will return in time. Don't be angry and wish things were otherwise – that serves only to tire the spirit and breed anxiety. Listen to music inside your home, read books, write – do things that feed the soul and calm the mind. When you are outside the home, feast your eyes on the beauty, find the joy. Fall back in love with things you had stopped looking at, or never found the time. All the other vexations of the universe outside will still be there when you are able to step outside your quiet universe once more. There will be cars on the road and clothes in the shops. The work will still be there, meetings to attend and events to plan. For now, take stock of your good fortune, whatever that may be, and choose to be happy. Find your own measure of gratitude and hold her close.

(2020)

'You are a child of the universe, no less than the trees and the stars; you have a right to be here. And whether or not it is clear to you, no doubt the universe is unfolding as it should….. With all its sham, drudgery and broken dreams, it is still a beautiful world. Be careful. Strive to be happy.'

Desiderata.

Found in the old Saint Paul's Church, Baltimore. Dated 1692.

How does it make you feel?

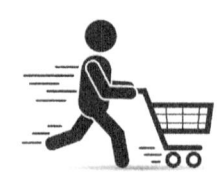

'No one ever forgets how you make them feel' … it's customer service 101. We used to do a lot of customer service training back in the day and that line always resonated with me.

I went into a small market to buy a few things. The lady behind the counter didn't even look at me. She took my money and slapped the change down on the counter. 'Have a good day!' I said, as I left. Nothing. I likely won't go into that shop again – she made me feel worse than when I went in. So many of us are in the customer service business in this world. Whether you are in real estate, banking, aviation or retail – the people in front of you, or over the phone, are your customers and they are helping to pay your salary. Please remember that – no matter what type of day you are having.

My relationship with the Salinas newspaper began on Halloween 1991, my first day of employment with them in the classified advertising department. This relationship grew over the years as I traversed the advertising departments into retail and real estate and finally into management. In the hay-day of newspaper, we would be out in the *field* visiting clients and come back to full page, full color ads on our desks – we were the king of our realm, top of the class. Everyone who was anyone had to be in the newspaper. Our building was large with copious staffing throughout – from the night press to the delivery personnel to the photographers, paste up crew, reporters, advertising. It was a live building 24/7 back then – a super fun and interesting place to work, no matter the pressures to make more and do more, that comes along with the territory of a large media monster with financial goals to make and exceed. I made some of my very best friends inside those inky walls and have some terrific memories.

I should have known the writing was on the wall when this pesky stuff called *direct mail* came along. We used to tell everyone it wasn't invited into the home like the local newspaper; it didn't have value like the paper that people paid for and looked forward to every day – or, in the case of the Salinas paper back then, 6 days a week. It's called *target marketing* – some of our advertisers argued back, as they switched from paper to direct mail and almost broke our hearts. Then the paste up and press crew got laid off and the press went quiet. Computers had come along and made the whole pre-press to press areas obsolete. It was a sad day when I went down to the basement and saw the old red press beast sitting there on her death watch. It was the end of an era.

But the old newsies battled on. Large departments became smaller, areas like *marketing* went away, there was some regional sharing of accounting and more. Some of us knew the business was heading the way of the dinosaur. Much as we loved our paper, the younger generation had these darn smart phones to read anything they might be interested in. They certainly did not want 'yesterday's news tomorrow,' as we would joke with each other. Circulation started to tumble, we weren't making our advertising targets, clients were not renewing contracts. We were at the beginning of a very desperate time in our industry. I got a position with another paper group and then quickly changed careers nearly 2 decades ago. I still wrote for the old paper on occasion and seemed to have a nice following of my column with the new group, but where would it go from here? How would we know who had died and what the local sports teams had done that weekend? We loved that old paper. Then the iconic building was closing its doors and the skeleton crew left behind were moving to a non-descript office close by. Outsourcing had taken over a lot of the live voices over the phone and I no longer knew who my ad rep might be.

Then the end of the line came in my relationship with the old gal. I had been a subscriber since 1991, when I was also an employee. That is nearly 3 decades of my life. One day, my paper just didn't arrive in my driveway. I emailed the circulation division and hoped it was just a glitch and it would show up eventually. Nope. Though the paper was now down to 3 days a week, I still looked forward to my little comfort time with the old broad. I still liked to drink my coffee and flick through. I tried to reach a live person to find out what the heck. Nope. I sent an email to whoever I could trace through the web site. I receive an email in return telling me that 'Your area is not deliverable. You have been canceled.' What? After 30 years of loyal service, just like that, I have been canceled? I was very upset. It was like being totally unfriended by one of your besties. I sent another email, since at least this prompted some kind of response. "Thank you for letting us serve you. You have been canceled." A few days later, I receive a portion of my outstanding annual circulation payment in the mail. No letter, no farewell, no 'thank you for reading all these years and please feel free to try and find a rack that works.' Nothing. There's customer service for you. I was unusually upset at this horrible treatment and pledged to tell anyone who would listen. My old newsie buddies just rolled their eyes, as if to say, 'what would you really expect?' All those years of customer training led up to being canceled by the operation I had been so loyal to and that rather hurt my feelings.

No, you never forget how someone makes you feel. I'm so glad that weekly papers still carry on serving their customers in their communities and I always know who my crew are and how to reach them. Too bad the media monsters never absorbed any of the customer service training modules they forced down our throats. They might have been able to do something clever to save the old lady.

(2021)

Joy Seeking

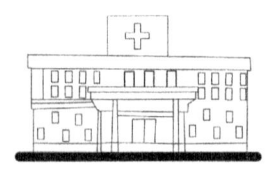

I couldn't think what to do with myself. My baby girl was lying in a hospital bed with a broken back, when she should have been enjoying the vacation of a lifetime in Montana. She was heavily drugged and monitored. She slept a lot in those early days. I spent a few restless night hours on the window ledge literally. There was a shortage of pillows in the hospital, so there wasn't one for me. It reminded me of what jail must be like. A narrow bench on the ledge of no hope. Her boyfriend stayed at her bedside with her. He and I both sported the largest black rings under our eyes like English badgers.

During the daytime hours, I was the gopher. "What do you want for lunch? Need a coffee? Any supplies you want from Target?" I tried to put the Practical into the hell that was those long, angry hours, when my daughter was at Kaiser Hospital in Vacaville and, as her mother, I wanted to just fix her and take her home. I also wanted to fix – in a manner of speaking – the person that did this to her. Who, in the so-called civilized world, drives on the wrong side of the freeway?

I had to use navigation everywhere I went during those days, because I was so sleep-deprived I had no brain to navigate a thing. The nearby Target nearly knew me by name. I went there to pick up toothpaste, drinks, whatever it seemed we needed in our cocoon of room 307. I would find myself mindlessly buying stuff to try and fill that gaping hole in my soul. Oh, here's a shirt she will like, a pair of shorts, a dress to wear under her back brace. I kept going back there in the hope that it would make all of us feel a little better with the senseless gifts that accompanied my return. I lost my car one day in the parking lot at the hospital. I walked round and round that enormous complex in well over 100-degree heat, only to find myself back near the entrance to the main building where I had – fall back in amazement – actually parked my car in a sensible spot.

Your senses are so enhanced when life throws you a curveball that you can no way catch; yet they are also numb and inhibited, sometimes ineffectual. Concerned folks would call me on the phone – I would be numb to the ring and miss their calls entirely. I was immune to the tick of the clock or the passing days. I found I didn't hardly have the energy to answer emails or texts. I had one goal in mind. I had to get my girl well enough to transport her home. Back to Target I would go, when the going got tough and it wasn't going to happen that day. Or the next day, apparently. I would be watching the sun in the sky, the dip of light, as it turned from early to later in the afternoon and I would know that she was gripped with terror and pain and wasn't going to be able to leave that day. It was a precious balancing act. She didn't want to get in the car. She was terrified to leave the sanctuary of Room 307. Personally, I wanted to just keep going back and forth to Target. That had become my own safety zone.

Once I finally managed to get her home, the depression kicked in a little and the fury rebounded in no uncertain terms. With the completion of the police report, so came the knowledge that the driver who hit her suffered from dementia, had no driving license and had been convicted of a similar wrong-way offense in 2019. Who had allowed this person to live freely on the streets; who gave her permission and a car to drive? The vehicle in the accident was fresh off a car lot with paper tags? The mind boggles.

In your efforts to do something positive, anything constructive, while the wheels of justice turn and the insurance procedures do their thing, you have to bring something fabulous to the table. In true animal-rescuer style, I brought kittens. "Which one do you want?" I asked Francoise and Aaron. "Ooh!" they squealed in their excitement that, finally, something nice was happening to them. "How about this one, how about that one?" They couldn't make up their minds. "Wait! What's better than one kitten? Two kittens!" I laughed, knowing that would take them over the edge with delight. So, two kittens it was, and Colter and Beaux arrived at Solace last week to great fanfare. The dogs just rolled their eyes as if to say, 'really?' They had been there before on the kitten train and knew it was quite the trip.

And then I started to think about the impacts of a nasty accident that was not your fault. You are not able to work or make money the way you normally do. Any disability payments that might come your way will take a while to process. You will still have all your regular bills in addition to medical. What could I do to make a difference there? Then I remembered the *Go Fund Me* efforts I had put together for other people; or, certainly, contributed to over time myself. People are often very generous with this type of thing, especially if it affects young people or animals, when they are in a difficult situation that was no fault of their own. During a sleepless night, it came to me that I would put together a *Go Fund Me* for the young ones and try to cheer their spirits; also make a few beans to help them out. And it did just that. I saw my daughter smile open-heartedly when she saw the generous spirits of near strangers reach out to them during their times of need. I saw hope in her big blue eyes that lifted my heart.

We may never know why a middle-aged woman with dementia was driving without a license on the wrong side of a freeway near Reading, causing this horrible accident that destroyed a young couple's dream vacation, truck and possessions – also broke my daughter's back. We can only control our response to the aftermath of this terrible incident and heed the reaction of those close to us and close enough to care.

In the depths of her disability and despair, my daughter was reminded that there are many good and generous souls out there. There is light outside her window. Though she is still practicing her walking and is a long way from driving a car or returning to work or school; in time we hope she will be okay, and her spirits will be good and restored and ready for better times ahead.

Thanks to all who have cheered Aaron and Francoise along their difficult journey. This Mama-Bear thanks you so much for all the love.

(2021)

My first impressions

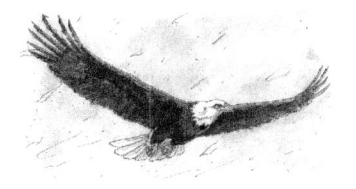

I've been living in America for 35 years now. Almost to the day. There you have it. I am either very old – or I came to this country very young – you be the judge of that. It is truly amazing how time flies and how I cannot believe I have lived in this country longer than in my home country of origin. That certainly puts things in perspective!

When I arrived in the US, I had not done my homework. I had no clue how things worked over here – it was all a mystery I found out mostly the hard way. We speak a similar language – kinda – but I found that even that is hard to navigate your way through at times, especially when there is a presumption it is the same language. (I do recall being asked on occasion if the primary language in England was French…?)

(Who calls their child Randy? How does Charles go to Chuck without it being funny? Why all the misspellings of perfectly well-spelled words? See favor, flavor, labor … or, more comfortably, favour, flavour, labour?) It is very hard to do anything or get anywhere in America, I discovered, if you had your formative base someplace else. (Regardless of whatever similarity of language.) I couldn't open a bank account with a certain large bank because I had no family banking history in the US (That's right, Einstein. I am a First-Generation Immigrant. They do happen.) I couldn't account for work experience because they didn't want to call for references overseas or trust that they would be accurate ones if they did. (See, again, do they speak French in England?) Everything was just super odd the first few months I lived over here. Okay, so, truthfully, the East Coast is a bit odd anyway – not a super fan – but I didn't know any better, so it was my landing point, a place to start. It could so easily have been the place I stopped and said never mind, fleeing home with all kinds of bad impressions in my wake.

When you just get off the boat, as it were, you are starting with a minus stature in this country. It was exciting initially to go to the grocery store and see 500 types of cornflakes or 25 different ways to envelop a chocolate biscuit with marshmallow; it was a blast to go through a drive through and imagine yourself back in the times of *American Graffitti,* those marsh-mellow days of great music, cars and style, now you were now in the heartland of all that; but that dairy wore off fairly sharpish, once reality kicked in – (don't ever go to the streets behind the

White House, they are a howling ghetto, shame on us) – it was hard to convince people of your authenticity, when they got all drunk over your accent. And they didn't know what a green card was and what it entailed. ("Are you Illegals? – No – you're citizens?" "No, again.") I was left with the blehs. Fortunately, my youthful ignorance/optimism made sure that I knew, in the back of my mind, I could return home at any time, that this could just be a curious stepping-stone from my former life to the new and improved one which was likely another step beyond the current land mass where I found myself. I didn't make friends, I didn't find any kindred spirits, the weather was dreadful – there really wasn't much good news to report, except my *illegal* job on Security at the State Department was a bit of a hoot. (You have to be a citizen to work there. I wasn't. Post 9/11, I believe that has now changed.) But then when I found out that their sense of humor (or more comfortably humour) was way different to ours, I recall thinking there was no way I would be able to stay. If you cannot find things funny, like ever, that is a bit of a game changer.

I can't exactly remember when I found *Seinfeld*. (Like finding God, but funnier.) I am not entirely sure; but I think it was likely about 2 years into this American adventure that is still going on and winding its way towards who knows what. I remember pausing at the comedy show before me. Wait, this was pretty funny! I sat down and watched some more. There was American comedy out there that would make me laugh? I felt as if I were stepping out of a cultural desert and into the light of a place where I might be able to stay a little while longer. I remember consciously deciding to look for that show again. I needed to make sure it really was funny; not a one-off. If I could trust that an American comedy show could make me laugh; then there was hope, real hope, that I just might be able to hang out in this rather extraordinary, cultural mishmash of an enormous land mass I had found myself in a bit longer.

The 1980's characters of Jerry, George, Elaine, Kramer – even Newman – made me feel more at home. I sought out the show to feel less homesick and more connected to the people and things around me. I never understood why, but other English friends of mine liked it too.

To this day, 35 years down the road, I still record the Seinfeld series and keep for when I'm feeling a little low, a tad shy from the touch of the laughter and friendship I miss from home, my original home. The characters from the show insert me into a universal level of regular life quirkiness and humor (or humour), that is like a welcome home song in my mind that embraces my senses and breeds a divine situ of contentment. Why does it remind you of home, you might ask. It's based in New York, not London? I don't know the answer to that exactly. What I do know is that my old friends – my Elaines, Jerrys, Kramer's and George's – have always been there in my life, my living room, supporting and cheerleading me through and onto the next adventure. With the techy aids of modern society and the diversity of communities the world over, New York is right there on a par with London, they are not so far away. Looking back at my first impressions of this country I have made my home; I am reminded how very similar we all are. We can speak the same language and be poles apart. We can share a similar language – or none at all – and yet be soul mates with the odd cultural challenge ahead. My first impressions reviewed 35 years later – aren't we lucky to live where we do?

(2023)

Nashvegas

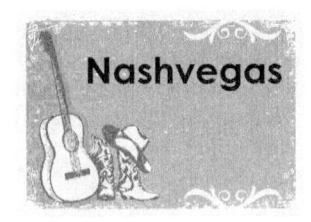

Ever since my sister passed, my daughter and I have been wont to follow her lead and give each other experiences instead of merchandise for special occasions. I was so delighted when the kid gave me concert tickets for Christmas. I love concerts, I adore music. We always have fun wherever we go. And then I paused. July? A summer concert in July in the deep South. I did know better. Having lived in Louisiana for 2.5 years, you never forget that kind of persistent, wet heat that springs moisture out of pores you didn't know you had. That kind of heat. I recall, not fondly, returning to England from Baton Rouge after another blistering summer. "Oh!" someone remarked. "But you are so white! I thought it was hot there?" Ha, yes, you stay inside during the long summer, I had to explain, and I still don't think they understood. No one ever truly understands the humidity of a deep-south summer unless they have experienced it first-hand. "Thank you so much, darling!" I said at the time, gulping. George Strait, how fabulous. In July. In Nashville. Weep.

I had wanted to go to Nashville for a very long time – it was totally on my proverbial list. So many of my favorite artists spring from this hallowed place. How could I not want to see some of America's greats in those famous halls?

I was packing for my trip to Nashville. Bathing suits, flip flops, sun dresses, hats, sunblock … was there anything else I might need? No, that would likely cover it. Oh, and some Skin-So-Soft for the bugs. I had visited Florida since my days in Louisiana, so the humidity wasn't going to be a surprise, was it.

The flight took us to Nashville via Dallas and was nicely uneventful. On the landing approach to Nashville, the pilot advised that all window blinds should remain closed due to the *heat advisory*. I had never heard of that! 'Please leave the blinds down when we land also,' he went on, 'Nashville is under a severe weather alert." Oh dear. I could only imagine. We found out super quick, as we called for an Uber to take us to our hotel and the wafts of boiling air hit us in the face. Immediately the sweat began to drip down the face. We drank water and still the sweat poured.

Arriving at the lovely Holston hotel at the top of Broadway was a delight. Lovely cool lobby, stylish temperate rooms, a pool at the top of the hotel with a city view and bar didn't hurt us one bit after the long day's travels. We took off downtown and witnessed the newly self-described *NashVegas* on a Thursday night. The streets were teaming with young things wearing next to nothing, bars packed, lines of people everywhere. Where was the music? You could hear a lot of it around, but there were too many people waiting to get through the door. What happened to the music? This all seemed to be about sex, drugs and alcohol. I dutifully showed my Id – ahem- and we enjoyed a couple of crazy drinks in the mix with too many others at the top of the Ole Red bar. We did get to visit with a few of the locals and found out that Californians were not too popular with their kind. I found that a bit strange, because people are people wherever you go – smart, ignorant and indifferent; but it seemed as if the political divide was as mind-blowing in Tennessee as it might be anywhere in our large land mass. That hadn't crossed my mind before we came. The old classic *Tootsies* bar where many a music great started their career was crowded; everything was overcrowded. We loved the lush coolness of the Glenn Campbell Museum and lamented that so few felt it was a priority, that the museum would be moving to smaller digs. The Willie Nelson Museum was equally stunning and entrenched in history – however most people were just hanging out in the gift shop. I do have to say that, almost without exception, the 'wait staff', bartenders and uber drivers were all superb and happy to see us.

The concert, however, was all about the music. Chris Stapleton and George Strait both kicked it out of the park. Though the arena was outdoors, with no misting or cool air for the crowd, it was 100 degrees and sweat-wet with humidity (never before have I actually poured ice cold water on my head and down the front and back of my dress) and it actually seemed to get hotter as the night progressed. There is something about live music that awakens a vital sense in your soul. It gives you something that nothing else can, no matter the weather. We were so lucky we went that night. The following night, the repeat concert was canceled due to the most incredible thunder and lightning storms I have witnessed in a while (from the sanctuary of my room!)

Perhaps the inclement weather was just an indication of the stormy travels we were to endure the following day, which was travel day. We were picked up at 3.45am and had a swift and successful trip to the airport. Bags were checked in without incident and we were soon sleepy-eyed at our gate well in advance of our 5.35am flight. Then the flight was pushed to 5.40, 6, 7, you get the picture. At the last check, it was postponed to 9pm at night; but we had already lost trust in them, (plus we had a connection we had already missed in Dallas), so we weren't going to be back in Cali that night if we hoped that they would deliver us there and many had work the next day.

We booked another flight at some cost from Nashville directly to San Francisco, securing the last 5 seats on the plane, and the first airline was forced to remove our bags from the hold once we made our request to cancel the flight (they also smashed up one of our bags). Our car was parked in San Jose, so we would have to Uber from San Fran to San Jose, but that was likely the only way we were going to get home that same night. The new flight was supposed to take off at 7pm and, at press time, it was pushed to 7.25pm. We still hope to get home tonight and that the airline gods that are watching over our skies will take pity on us poor travelers who have now spent around 15 hours – or a flight to China – in the airport.

If you read the recent travel news, it has been quite the ugly summer for some American airlines. With canceled flights and passengers dumped all over the place, I have now added another corporation to the no-good airlines I shall never again fly with. "Here's a number you can call and try to get a refund," the 'Customer Service' lady told us. I highly doubt that suggestion was even worth the cost of the long and frustrating phone call that would ensue with no good result. (We eventually arrived home at 1am. It had taken us nearly 24 hours to get home from Nashville.)

NashVegas, huh. It will be a while before I go back. If ever.

(2023)

On the circuit

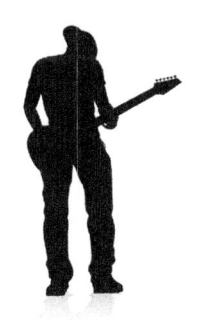

I've been on the tour circuit these past couple weeks. Not like a rock star tour circuit, but a circuit of sorts. For those of you who know me, you know I'm a writer not a speaker, so this concept has been a little against my grain. But it's good to stretch yourself, however old, right? Teaching an old dog new skills and all that.

My friend is on the *Impower* board. *Impower* is a superior organization, powered by go-getting women who work to get professional people together to engage, visit, share bread, listen to a – hopefully– interesting speaker and invest in local non-profits in our community. I knew that already. They also put together a nice lunch at attractive sites for those of us who like to, on occasion, cross the lettuce curtain.

"What are you doing on October 14?" my friend asks me with some anxiety in her voice. (She's on the Impower board). "I'm going to Impower," I tell her. "YOU ARE??" (Well, yeah, I go when I can.) "Our Olympian speaker can't make it," she tells me. "Will you speak?" When someone asks you a difficult question like that and you don't want to disappoint, but you don't like public speaking, things go a little blurry. "Ummmm. I guess I could do that," I respond mumbly and meekly. And then I promptly forgot about it. Until I didn't. I woke up in the middle of the night with a jump. I had to be engaging and amusing, also interesting, in front of maybe 70-100 people for about 40 minutes. This was a challenge when I really thought about it. Then I went on vacation. I return home from Europe and realize my speaking gig is in 2 days, no pressure. This crowd wasn't one where you could wing it. I started practicing, trying not to umm too much, or creepily laugh at all my own jokes.

It was a glorious day, the morn of my big speech. The aim in these situations is to be on site nice and early. It eases any nerves and situates one near perfectly for the performance ahead. We did just that at the lovely Pasadera Country Club off Highway 68. And then old friends started showing up and I realized that this was actually going to be really fun. I wasn't as rehearsed as one might hope to be under these circumstances, but hey, I had done some acting in my time and these people weren't going to be rude and boo me, at least, were they? After all, many were my friends. I warned the crowd that they had been previously offered a full refund for the tickets they had purchased for the Olympian, and they had chosen not to cancel at the time; so, they were stuck with me for the next half hour. They laughed! That is always a good start. I just chuckled a little, not a full belly-laugh with mouth wide open – a small, respectable chuckle. I started to find my groove. This speaking gig was not so bad.

In fact, in retrospect, it was a delightful event, and I had a really good time. I got to visit with friends I hadn't seen in a while, I sold some of my books and I helped raise money for a wonderful cause. There was even a miniature pony there from the elected charity, for crying out loud. (No, they didn't let me take him home!) Want me as a public speaker? Yeah, I have some experience of that. I *do* circuits, apparently.

Next, it was the tea circuit in Soledad – a popular joint fundraiser for the South County Animal Rescue and the Soledad Historical Society, as was a few years back. The last tea party was pre-pandemic, so it had been a while. Here I was onsite with two water kettles and 2 large tea pots on the go, numerous jugs of milk, English tea bags and sugar in addition (note to self, 3 kettle and tea pots might be a good idea next time. That crowd was hard to keep up with!) Tea, sandwiches, cookies and cakes were served with the tea. Folks were able to select their own china teacup and saucer when they entered, and, fortunately, young folk from the 4H and the Aztecs Track Team were there to assist in all necessary things, including the pouring of the boiling hot English tea. (Please don't burn anyone, I begged them!) It was a decent event and well attended. Hopefully some money was made for both organizations, because that's the whole idea! At the end of the afternoon, I could barely even walk, let alone talk. That tea-pouring gig is hard work!

From the tea circuit, it was onto the 1st Annual fundraiser for the Cattlewomen's Association, (who knew that 2.5 cows constitutes eligibility to be a member!) so kinda like a Rodeo circuit? (Fortunately, no one asked me how many head of cattle I owned, since 2.5 might be a dead giveaway – Insert Random Cowboy: "You mean 2500 head?") They accepted LUNAbooks, my personal book shop, as a vendor at their event at the Monterey Fairgrounds and I was so proud of this branching out from my comfort zone of fundraising for other entities or just giving the darn things away. I was actually, to coin a phrase, 'getting out there' …

I tell you, this 'getting out there' business is a lot! My friend helped me set up all the stuff at the Fairgrounds on Friday. (First you had to actually find the place, locate the spot where you unload, schlepp the boxes, unpack the boxes and all that good stuff! It was a work-out!) Then we had to come up with a decent display and figure out all we were missing. Then we had to go shopping to combat our fatigue and fulfil our retail stress for the week!

Bright and early the next morning, I was off to find my booth at the Fairgrounds, armed with vital items I was missing from my display, and hopefully enough sleep onboard to get me through the day. It was going to be a long day, 12-8pm, and we all hoped for mega crowds to keep us busy. The crowd thing didn't really materialize, but it wasn't a bad showing and, though a super longgg day, I did sell 10 books and met some new people. So, getting out there on various circuits is quite time-consuming and maybe not very lucrative, but it does make for an interesting life. As my clever husband duly noted, if you don't want to 'get out there' (that takes days of your life to accomplish) just print enough books for a few friends and family and don't even worry about it. The jury is out on that, but I did some pretty good circuits these last few days and, truth be told, I am beat.

(2023)

The 48-hour blackout

You would have thought the end of the world was nigh, or at least we were at the beginning of a very long siege where everyone would be marooned in darkness in their homes. The grocery store was like armagedon with empty shelves, lines of people anxiously looking at their smart phones, carts piled up with batteries, matches, water and the like. "I don't think the power will go off here," said the trusty check out dude. And I didn't think so either. It was like being under a tornado watch. "Supposed to happen at 5pm." Nope. Missed us. "Supposed to be 7pm. No wait, 8 …"

After 8pm came and went, I felt quite smug in my comfy home with all my lights and accoutrements around me. We had underground power lines after all;' what kind of risk would our area have? I watched the evening news with those poor folks and their animals evacuating from fire-ravaged areas, followed by conversations with more local mountain folk who were already in a black out situation so to speak. I think the fire folk were a little more accepting in some ways. At least they could see the fires and/or smell the smoke.

Finally, at about 10.45pm we were firmly in the dark with alarm clocks flashing and the like. I had not even dug out the flashlights from last year's daylight savings time, let alone looked for batteries to put inside them. I just didn't think it would happen. Oh well, as I turned over in my cozy shelter. At least it was nighttime. Maybe the power would be back on tomorrow. The morning came and no power. We searched through the utility app on the smart phone to see if there was any update. "Yes, you are currently in a no-power zone," it informed us helpfully with no end in sight.

All of a sudden, I was in panic mode. Not because I didn't have batteries or provisions or whoever knows what you might need if the power is out for days on end. No, this was a critical emergency – today was a 49er game and we had no power! This was time to call out the emergency troops, the National Guard even. We would have no Sunday football at our house – and the television wouldn't tape it either. I cast around for places to go, people to call., Fortunately, my friend and neighbor had been preparing a lot better than us. "Wanna come over for the game?" she asked. They had a powerful generator that would power many things, as well as a couple of televisions for the game. Oh boy, I could breathe again. "How do I get through your gates?" I ask her. Silence. Hadn't prepared that far.

The strange day then continued, as I found myself clambering over walls and she driving through vineyards and fields to pick me up since we didn't know how to get her gates opened without power. And what fun we had. The game was made even more entertaining by the camping out feel to it; not to mention the wonderful camping snacks and wine. Sometimes you have to get out of your comfort zone to realize just how lucky you are.

Meanwhile back at the house, the Mother-in-law was sitting depressed and bereft in her chair, no tv to watch, no heater to put on. I told her to get out of her chair and into the sunshine where she would likely feel a lot better. She refused to eat anything in the fridge since it had likely already spoiled. "You're spoiled," I felt like saying to her. But nothing was going to burst my bubble on the day the 49ers won again, and I got to enjoy the game, even though there was no power at my house.

A message came in from our homeowner association telling us to conserve our water. Oh yes, we need power for our water pumps too. Our gates wouldn't open, we couldn't wash any clothes or boil any water. There were no regular lights in the house and – gosh darn it – some of us couldn't watch any television.

Finally, Monday afternoon we were rescued from our *misery* – though it was more than usually peaceful at my house – and plunged back into the work of all we could not do the days we had no power.

How lucky we are to live in a world where, mostly, everything is at your fingertips. I just couldn't find much of a reason to complain. If I had been up in the fire areas, I would have appreciated the small concessions from others, that the fire fighters might be able to focus on the fires at hand, without others adding to the mele. I'm hoping it helped some. Though the conversations will likely continue for some time as to how a State like California should not have to resort to rolling black outs during fire season, I had quite a fun weekend *camping out* and being able to do absolutely no work at all. Plus, did I mention, the 49ers won. Again.

(2019)

The Atmospheric River

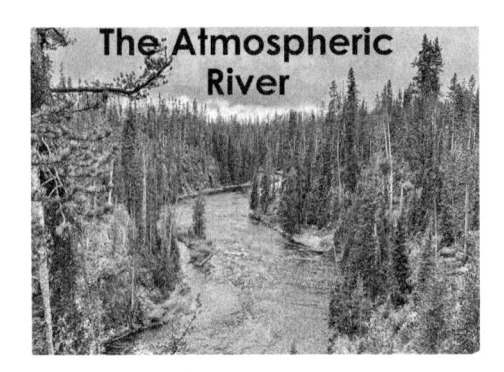

I love this time of year, when the *storm window* opens, the water possibilities increase ten-fold, and the population of our desiccated West Coast becomes transfixed by weather and all her whims. "We are on the storm watch", the forecaster whispers in spooky tones. We tune in just to see if we missed anything from the broadcast an hour ago. "Breaking News!" (Yes, by all accounts, we did!) "Get ready for potentially historic rainfall!" (Ooooh, historic! Love historic!) "Evacuation warnings are in place for the burn scar areas (Oh dear). Watch out for debris flows. Leave now!" These broadcasts take on an almost thriller aspect, much more interesting than your daily news banter about politicians caught doing naughty things and the movements of the Dow Index. No, this is non-judgmental stuff we can all get our teeth into on the West Coast, soon to be called the 'Wet Coast'. "The Atmospheric River is approaching the California coast, leave now! Flash flood warnings in place!" (Say it quickly.) Oh, I do love an Atmospheric River when she comes to visit. Though, truthfully, our State can never handle one of those spectacles when they pass us by. They always lead to flooding and all of the above described drama-rama; but it is so delicious to see our browns quickly turn to light greens, our weather forecasters talking about something other than the drought and the 2nd driest year on record, along with photo shoots of earnestly depressed politicians standing in dry river beds. It is so refreshing! There is also absolutely no cross-over between Covid and an Atmospheric River – even more fabulous!

Last winter was a complete wash-out – or rather dry-out – in the world of the water tables. It was pathetic. I honestly wonder why some of the geniuses of the world could not put their heads together and pipeline some of that gorgeous wet stuff from up north or wherever to our bone-dry State. We could do a trade for lettuce or broccoli, or even marijuana for goodness sakes. Would that be so hard to accomplish? Maybe, instead of taking a rocket up to Jupiter, they could spend a few gazillions on that project and stop all the stressful chaos every year. Yes, pretty much every year. You no longer hear much about desalination successes. We know it is possible, we know it is expensive. Make it less expensive for crying out loud. Let's take the salt out of the salt water and, lo and behold, we would have water we could use! Such a concept. Anyone listening, anyone?

Back to the Atmospheric River topic, because I just like saying it so much. My father in the British Isles, where it rains pretty much 7 out of every 10 days, giggles when I say that, because everyone knows California is such a dry state and we love to overreact when we are talking about a little bit of rain. You wait; the schools will likely be closed tomorrow, and the excited newscasters will be telling everyone to stay off the roads. People will be driving into ditches and power poles likes there's no tomorrow, because obvs they miss the memo time and time again that, it's finally raining, the roads are slick; it would be smart to drive less foolishly. Still, you will witness the foos hitting the 101 Northbound at commute time, driving right up the biosky of the car in front. You will see the make up being applied in the fast lane and the odd texter maneuvering the puddles to send that one vital message. Makes me crazy! Oh and then, of course, there will be the obligatory power outage with no end in sight.

I learned to drive in rain, snow, sleet and black ice. I'm not bragging; it was just a fact of the winters where I grew up. I also learned how to exercise double the caution, drive into a skid, apply only mild brakes – you know that kind of thing. So that when the Atmospheric River would hit – like often – I would be well-skilled at driving that death machine under those conditions. Might be also good for the smarty pants in the world, whilst they are pondering my other suggestions, to devise a driving program where people actually learn to drive in different conditions, because not everyone was born with common sense, apparently.

It is not always warm and dry in California, contrary to what myths might be concocted in that regard. We do have rain – normally not enough – we do have storms and – boy oh boy – when we are really lucky, we might get into that fabulous storm window we do rain dances for; not to mention the weather forecaster heaven when the storms stack up off the coast, ready to come and flood our glorious state; also throw us an Atmospheric River once in a while. We love the storm windows; we get so excited about them we can hardly stand ourselves. The dogs look up with concerned eyes at the billowing grey clouds and swirling winds. They beg to come in though it is neither cold nor wet; just weird. The doves fly by all wonky on the wind and even the flies are desperate to come in out of the storm window and rest a little while in the dry. It is so funny to witness.

Meanwhile, the Salinas River is still bone dry and we have received just a few small droplets on our patio. I haven't seen the sun today, but that's okay because it's laundry day and a day for indoor pursuits. I shall not be rushing out the door at dumb-commute time tomorrow either, because I know the sort of trouble that could be asking for. I shall be watching the weather and the traffic reports and tut-tutting over the latest person to skid into a ditch or the flooding that will inevitably happen on 101 North at Spence Road.

Idiocy is doing something more than once, when it didn't work out the first time. Some of our State's responses to water, or the lack therof, are simply idiotic. Pipeline, people! We need a water pipeline from the wet states to the dry ones. Could someone please drag Jack Genius off his next flight to Mars and have him devise something really smart in that regard?

Meanwhile, it's back to my Atmospheric River. Must be time for another weather update. Time to tune in. Wait, there's no power …

(2019)

The Coronation and other important news

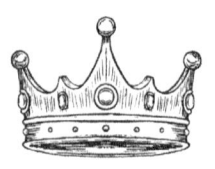

I was, coincidentally, in England right after the death of Queen Elizabeth. It was a most strange and eerie time in the country. The nation was in mourning well after the nation was officially mourning, as it were. I happened to walk along the Mall to Buckingham Palace at night, when all the barricades were still up and the roads blocked off. Flowers were littering the roadway and the palace looked grey and vacant, sad and lost.

I was again in the United Kingdom for the Coronation of King Charles III – less coincidental, truthfully, since I always come over to the UK for father's birthday and, this time, it happened to cross over with the coronation. As one monarch passes, the heir to the throne takes their rightful place in succession – a near seamless passing of the traditional gauntlet in these parts over hundreds of years. And yet, it didn't feel seamless, since Elizabeth had been the only monarch most of us ever knew – her passing felt like the death of a beloved Granny, and I know many, many people who were surprised by her death (she had looked so good the day before, all made up in her twinset and her pearls!) The Nation grieved heavily at her passing.

This did not feel the same. Were people turning away from the monarchy, looking for change in all the right places? Was the universally half damp reaction to King Charles heralding a change in the importance and direction of the Royal Family? I did wonder.

I wandered into the tourist shop at the airport, hoping to find a nice Coronation mug for father. There was one available – a rather quiet one in a muted color. I found this a bit surprising. You could still find souvenirs of Queen Elizabeth and even the Prince and Princess of Wales; but for the Coronation that was happening just around the corner, there was very little. At least the cup was made in England, I thought to myself, as I forked out the 22 pounds at the cash till.

It became clear that Father very much wanted to watch the Coronation that was being televised from early to quite late on May 6. Sister said she would put it on the TV for a bit and I soon found myself absolutely riveted by the pomp and circumstance. The immaculately groomed and bedecked horses and carriages paraded out of the courtyards of Buckingham Palace and along the Mall, as regally as they ever did. The King and Queen consort were escorted by the appropriate Guards in a gold carriage, a gift from the Silver Jubilee in 1977 apparently. Despite the drizzle, everything was bright and sparkly, the mood on the streets one of good humor and happiness. I had forgotten how well the English do these things. At Westminster Abbey, heads of State, Kings, Queens, Prime Ministers and more were welcomed to the 1000-year-old abbey. I enjoyed watching all the visitors who came to pay their country's respects in all manner of shapes, colors and hats. The choir boys were as delightful as the gospel singers. It really was quite a fun party, wrapped in oodles of historical ceremony and delicious diversity. The few minutes I had planned to spend watching the occasion quickly turned into hours. I missed the actual crowning of the King and had to revisit on Messers Google a bit later – but I have to say I really enjoyed watching the best of the British at work. I came away a little heartened by the wonderful procession and occasion that it might rather serve to solidify the relationship of the Royal Family with the world and remind all of us that theirs are wonderful and deeply established traditions that will be going nowhere in a hurry. I imagine I may yet see another Coronation in my lifetime! Who knows.

Of course, my most favorite part was the clinking, clanking and most beautifully dressed horses, especially the naughty greys. That's always my favorite part.

Randomly, in other news, I got to visit some other gorgeous horses this week, as my inaugural visit to the Isle of Man Home for Old Horses was on the agenda. I had been wanting to visit this special place for some time. The rescue sanctuary was founded in the 1950's for retiring dram horses (shires) that were an important part of the Douglas promenade scene, as they pulled carts of tourists back and forth along the seafront. These days, the home also embraces pit ponies and other equines in need of rescue. The lush meadows and wonderful staff made me so happy I had paid them a visit. I spent some money in their café and gift shop and fed carrots and apples to the old souls, including some very fun donkeys I would like to have shipped back to California. I shall return again soon, and most definitely over the holiday season when Christmas cards and other goodies can be purchased, and the home is bedecked with cheer.

In further Commonwealth news, father turned 94 this week and how amazing is that. We had a nice dinner out in his honor, we enjoyed tea and cake in the sun, and we will enjoy yet another favored cake on the actual day. I managed to find a nice china piece in a junk shop for him – the coronation of Edward VIII in 1937, when dad was only 8 years old. He was talking about that day only today – the third Coronation of his lifetime. I expect he will use it for his olive pips.

With all the horses I enjoyed observing, and birthdays and coronations that occurred this week, it has really been a wonderful several days.

"We are steeped in irony as a nation, and we wear our patriotism and loyalty privately and secretively. I love the way it bursts out for royal occasions. An extraordinary fluorescence, then it's gone."

Potter, Emma Bridgewater.

(2023)

Unmasked and Unaware

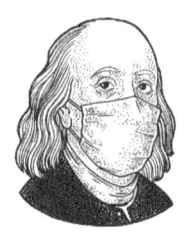

I had always been pretty proud of us. From the moment we were able, we were off to the pharmacy! Another shot? Yes please. With all the horror stories and truths from 2020 still fresh in everyone's minds, we did not want to get caught out by life, by being late, by standing a chance of contracting the C plague. And then it came to pass that the coronavirus pandemic no longer legally existed. You did not have to wear masks in government buildings or doctor's offices. It was over. We all signed a collective gasp of relief.

It wasn't so long ago that I asked my pharmacist about the next vaccine. Surely there would be one coming up, just around the corner? If there was one to be had, I wanted it. Regardless of any aftereffects of the jab, it was so worth it. He replied that there would 'likely' be one in the fall, so I left with a rather false sense of security. No one required masks on planes anymore, people barely remembered to carry the hand sanitizer they vowed would forever take a firm position inside their handbag. We were through; free and clear.

On the return trip from Nashville, one of our party said they weren't feeling well. Seemed like a hearty reaction from our less than fun return journey of diabolical flight cancellations and stress, or perhaps a touch of the flu from all the wild extremes in temperature we had experienced over the weekend, not to mention wild people. No one thought it might be you know what. Heading home after our mammoth travel day, it was well past midnight, I was the driver, and I was tired and thirsty. Everyone else was asleep. There was a water bottle right there and I drank out of it.

You can probably tell where I am going with this. Yes. Just a few hours later and I was swiftly going down with the modern-day plague. It's frighteningly all a bit of a blur, but I do know it hit me like a freight train and yelled in my pounding ear 'Yoo Hoo! Hadn't actually gone anywhere! So glad I get to visit with you for a while!' I was tired, sweaty, my head pounded, my ears were ringing, and the symptoms were all lined up right there for the little white stick to give me a positive result. Twice. After 3 years of avoiding its clutches, here I was in the midst of my own little coronavirus hell. It reminded me of chemotherapy that I had endured years ago. That weird weighty, out of body and mind feeling, the lack of taste and smell, the overwhelming fatigue that sat on you and made you sleep some more. My doggies loved it. Mummy was home and she was pretty much crashed out in her night-night all day and night! Mummy, on the other hand, kept trying to be useful to the world, do her work, complete her banking, unpack from her trip, but she couldn't. It was a most pitiful sight.

Husband kept taking my temperature – high, higher, high – for several days, administering solicitous Tylenol and ice-cold water as fever reducer helpers and approaching all masked up and with caution tape strapped around his head lest the Stupid-CoronaVirus, as our granddaughter used to call it, really was a lurgy that might be poised to physically attack and overcome, like a super monster.

In my rare moments of lucidity, I found myself cursing the lack of data on this latest strain that had attacked little moi in the deep south and ridden home on my back. Why were we not advised to be all masked up in 150-degree heat (that would have gone down real well!) since they don't believe in masking down there, let alone – much of the time – the existence of a real pandemic, I know that wouldn't have worked at all, but I would like to have had the opportunity to make my own choices about the matter. "Fully vaccinated and why am I getting this?" (Might as well say 'let's talk about my naked body' or something equally personal. I would have taken an extra shot, I would have double masked. Anything not to lose a week of my life in my bed with severe (think chemo) night sweats where the bed covers are drenched, hallucinogenic dreams (again chemo drugs) and foggy brain. Lack of taste or appetite except for well-buttered toast (shall I say chemo yet again?) Oh, my word, I shall need some serious post cancer treatment therapy after this little lot, and I haven't stepped foot in a chemo lab since 2010!

If you want to get all smarty pants about it and see where the super spreader stuff might be going on or where the upticks are – info that we used to be able to glean in a micro-second, the data is no longer reliable because testing is not being reported anymore. We are not in a pandemic, so this little burst of hell, for want of a better description, is largely due to my overactive imagination, my dislike for some of the things I witnessed in the deep south and my PTSD from chemo.

Zinc! They say! Get a hold of Paxlovid! Sleep, sleep, sleep (Yeah, not helpful!) Water, water, water! (Yes, I'm on that!)

When you know better in life, you do better, or so they say. This I now know. I shall be wearing masks on the plane for the rest of my life, so I had better invest in some comfy ones. I will do an immune system boot camp before I go anywhere ever again. I will never drink out of a suspect water bottle ever again. I will never again forget that coronavirus is still present in our communities, whether we like it or not and whether anyone is counting. Should you not want to be plagued like me for several days of your life with this affliction, check with your pharmacist as to when you can get another vaccine and wise up as to travel to – ahem – busy places. I wish I had read this story before my last adventure. I'm hoping that, in the writing of it, I shall feel a little less ripped off and more inclined to fight these awful symptoms and get back to my real life.

  PS I am still alive. I did, however, manage to successfully give the bug to husband. Fortunately, I was able to secure some Paxlovid for him and his symptoms were much milder than my own. Also, I read that there is quite the uptick in cases. A new strain they are calling Eerie, or something like that.

(2023)

Writing another book

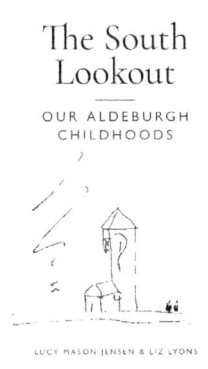

The South Lookout
OUR ALDEBURGH CHILDHOODS

LUCY MASON JENSEN & LIZ LYONS

I've heard it's as addictive as heroin; or even getting tattoos. Maybe it won't kill me, though sometimes I do wonder. Why do I do this to myself? I have a job; I have passions and a busy life. I don't know what it is, but for some reason I have to write. I've been writing ever since I knew how to and it doesn't seem to be stopping any time soon.

Writing itself is fine. Get a notebook, knock yourself out. No one has to get hurt. It can be really therapeutic. Even my weekly column is pretty unpainful and keeps my fingers a little busy and my brain ticking over. Times I have thought about stopping the weekly deadline madness and have missed the odd week or two in the paper, I will get messages that encourage me to keep writing, that people want to hear what I have to say, for whatever reason. People tell me they feel as if they know me – not sure if that is a good thing or not – even if we have never met.

I started writing newspaper columns when I was working at the Salinas paper, so somewhere around the happy days of newspaper publication in the early to mid-90's. Next, I did some reporting – less fun than the column – but better paid. Following that, it was back to a column when we moved down to South Monterey County, and I wanted to be a part of the local community. That means it is about two decades that I have been writing a column for this paper group. That's a lot of paper! And a lot of words.

I published my first book in 2011, named after my column *Window on the World*. It contained about 10 years of columns in some sort of topical order. I was super naive about self-publishing – still am – and purchased a rather expensive service to do the lot – from dealing with my manuscript to rolling print copies off the press. I think I'm still rather in recovery from that little adventure. But, being British, we are a stubborn lot and I had quickly forgotten about the battle scars of the first adventure in publishing and soon wanted to write a story about my beloved horse Winston, titled *Winston Comes Home*, a short, children's story illustrated with my own photos. I thought it was rather a beautiful story – also true. It finally appeared sort of how I had planned; but I was further disappointed by the whole self-publishing gig. Let's face it, you are not going to make much money out of this infliction of self-torture, this written word affliction that some of us suffer from; but it's tough trying to negotiate the fees and add-ins and pad-ins that some of the so-called *self-publishing* companies want to add to the cost of you being able to say 'there we go, finished with that one … just in time for the Christmas buying season, ha ha …yeah, get it on Amazon!' We are not allowed to say this, but I'm going to anyway. Kindle and e-books are a wonderful thing for the reader, a stupendous invention by some techy whizz kid who has never published a book in their lives and has made it so that when an author *sells* an e-book, basically the author will end up owing them. It's a necessary service; I get that, much I am of the tactile generation that cannot get along with e-readers and has to hold a printed book in my hand to really enjoy it; but, from the e-book, know this – the author gets almost zilcho for all their hard work.

Which brings me to my current adventure that was supposed to be completed just in time for last Christmas' buying rush … and is still a work in progress. I had various excuses last year not to be able to get her to the church on time, as it were. But then what happens over time is that you keep picking up and putting down the pieces of book, keep editing and re-editing stories until you are so sick of the darned thing you couldn't care less. I could hear my sister Rosie's voice in my head, however. "Oh c'mon sis, just get it done! You will feel so much better!" And she is, of course, right. I would be furious with myself if I abandoned all this hard work just because I'm bored of it. So, I started making maneuvers towards the finish line. I wouldn't go the same route as the last couple of times. I would get someone to paginate the tome for me and then figure out the rest.

All of a sudden, terms like *epub* and *mobi* start flying around. "Umm, can I also get it printed into … you know … like paper, once I have done all of this?" The assumption with these young techs is that you are only interested in an ebook, which, as a paper person, is a bit alarming. Though that may be the way some would choose to read my labor of love and definitely the cheaper way for the reader, you can't sign an *epub* or a *mobi* and I would definitely want hard copies printed for my readers who are more like me. Those who still want to pick up a newspaper in the morning and read a good old-fashioned paper novel in the bath.

Taking this new route to completion makes me rather nervous, I can tell you, my audience, that; but I'm hopeful the young tecchies will be kind and the literature gods aligned to ensure that this book does get published in e-book, mobi and the other way. And that I will be able to bring it to you, my best readers, right in time for the busy holiday buying season.

Thanks for always taking the time to read good stuff, especially the paper kind!

Lucy.

(2019)

SECTION 4

Me & Them

Introduction to –
Me & Them

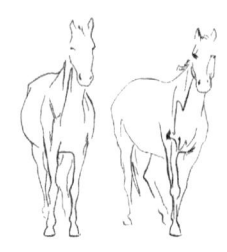

This is another spicy mish-mash of stories about me and them – me and the rescue horses, (yes, I have another one), me and my battle to be more like *them*, (people who practice yoga for example), me and the competition out there in the workplace, (what competition? Ha!). This section contains stories about the circumstances in life that make you either laugh, cry or go stir-bonking crazy. The times you think something is a good idea and then, five minutes in, you realize it is the worst idea ever and you are miles away from being able to make it right. The multiple plans you have for the week and then life comes along with other ideas and puts you to bed. The day your credit card gets hacked, and you spend most of the day trying to figure out the charges and how the heck … then you have to call all of the auto charges that will be coming out of the now defunct card and wait for ages trying to talk to a human, sigh. Those wasted hours we spend on the necessary minutiae of life. You know – that stuff.

And then the beautiful stories that combat the tales of chaos and minutiae in daily life like Andrew and his gorgeous Labs (one black and one yellow) that took over the Internet when we needed them to, or the inspiring young people that worked at the local expo and took all my books home for free because they told me they loved reading.

Me & Them is like life itself, a rollercoaster ride of how you successfully navigate this life, and nobody gets hurt. How to be almost always consistently patient and kind. How to embrace what you love and tolerate what you don't. Or do your best with all of the above? I am sure you will recognize yourself in this section and the testing of your sanity that happens quite often to the occupants of the modern world,

Like them? Let me know – lucymasonjensen@gmail.com

Tony, Mary and me

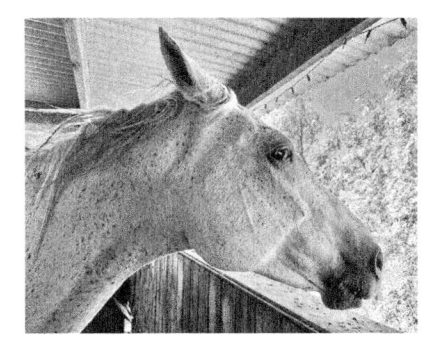

During the last several months of covid – or lifetime – depending on how you feel about it; people and animals have become even closer, I've noticed. Record adoption levels at shelters were noted the world over. People now needed an excuse to walk the dog, they wanted to walk the dog and get away from the prison that used to be their home with all their so-called beloveds inside. Maybe not everyone felt that way, but I know many who told me that being allowed to exercise their dog during the covid lock down became a habit which became an essential part of their everyday, lock down or not. I was afraid that the shelters would then start filling up again once people returned to work and regular life, but, thus far, it doesn't seem that way. It appears as if the animals have become a much more intrinsic part of your average household; more civilizing than many of the family members in some cases. A lot of us already knew that about animals; it took a worldwide pandemic to teach some of the late starters.

Olive and Mabel are two Labradors who own a man called Andrew Cotter. If you do not already know about Olive and Mabel, you have been living under a rock these past covid-ridden months. What is special about these Labradors, you might ask! Well, truthfully, absolutely nothing; but they are just so delightful as most dogs are. Their dad Andrew is a British sportscaster who found himself a little unemployed and, let's face it, skint – to coin a nice English turn of phrase that means broke – during the pandemic. He started to do voice-overs for the Labs and became an internet sensation. Why, you might ask! Well, one reason is he is very funny and the other is that he totally understands dogs and their patterns of thought. That for dog people is an essential part of life. Who knew that such a *talent* would turn viral almost overnight and have people going to *YouTube* just to see what kind of food-seeking and mountain climbing the Labs were going to do next. Good for Andrew is what I say and when is the movie coming out? (Oh, a movie about dogs and food-seeking and mountain climbing, you might roll your eyes! Yes, with Mabel and Olive and Andrew and these are very fun characters to spend some time with.) Though Andrew may not yet have made his fortune with his overnight sensation, he likely at least gets a free year of kibble that promotes his lovely Labs or has some mountain climbing gear sponsorship. (Oh, but wait, he wrote the books too – and those likely made him pretty comfortable in life! I bought the books for myself and my doggy friends!) And, noteworthy, he didn't even do it for the money; he did it for the love of his dogs and his own sanity, it seems.

Moving on from that topic, but not really at all; I must introduce you to the horses of Riverview – or ponies as my father and aunt insist upon calling all splendid specimens within the equine world – I wonder how viral their lives might go in the scheme of things. They were raised on an unsuitable *ranch* of sorts close by to our neighborhood. Tony, as the colt is called, was born rather unceremoniously in the neighboring vineyard when his mother Mary, yes, bolted through the broken-down fence – no barbed wire, thank you lord – and gave birth in the middle of nowhere. Thanks to some worried vineyard workers, she was coaxed back to the *ranchita* with her baby. It could have ended up really badly. Things on the *ranchita* went from bad to worse. Many of our neighbors have stopped by and checked on the water and food status of the horses, since it seemed to be unreliable at best. Too many times I drove past and witnessed the horses car-watching and seemingly waiting for an owner that never seemed to come. One time I called the landlord of the property and told him I was going to cut the lock on the gate and do a well-check on the animals. It was 100 degrees outside and, sure enough, the horses – and the dog at the time – had no food or water. I was absolutely beside myself, rectified the situation and drove to the man's house to give him a piece of my mind. He was too scared to face me that day, but at least the animals got fresh food and water. The situation continued to decline from there and one of our neighbors got his permission to rescue the horses and bring them closer to home where we could properly take care of them, Mary, the Mare, was super slim and the colt slim and skittish. I think they were rescued just in time, before some serious ailments assaulted them. Our neighbor with the nice corral and stalls volunteered her 'pasture' for them. Other neighbors helped pitch in with food and supplies. Alfalfa, apples, grains, beet pulp and fresh water was delivered to these animals. They must have thought they had gone to heaven. The Mama Mary is sweet with kind eyes and, obviously, a lovely nature. She reminded me of my old Winston and brought tears to my eyes as I brushed her and remarked upon her relaxed poise with the tip of her back hoof resting gently on the ground. Winston would always do that when he felt secure.

Who knows where these innocent animals will end up; but at least, for now, they are well-fed and watered and safe. And, as for Olive and Mabel, they are absolutely living the life, as all animals should, with their lovely Andrew.

(2020)

Bad days, a new book and sailing around the world

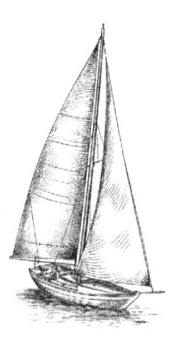

It was simply one of those days. A wake-up call that didn't involve coffee or soft music, let alone the sound of little birds singing to herald the dawning of a new day. "This is Bank of America. We have reason to believe that your credit card has been compromised…" Oh, blooming great. The one we use for all the household stuff, our go-to, the one that gains us all those precious air miles. Yes, that one. "Madam, did you happen to purchase tickets for the New York ballet?" No, I did not. Masterful how they flag some things and not others. I don't look like a ballet fan, perhaps? A few days away from our European vacation and this gives me a sore head right at the beginning of the day. "Can they just move all the auto-charges from this card to the other one?" I plead with Fraud Department in my sweetest little girl English voice. "Oh no, Ma'am. You have to make all those calls yourself." Of course, you do.

Then the escrow that was supposed to be closing in a matter of a few days started to crumble to its knees and there the money I had already spent, likely sitting, as we speak, on that coveted credit card, was not to be ….right in the heart of the Christmas shopping season. That was annoying too. Whoosh and all that work was gone.

Where was my other card? You know that other one that I don't normally use. That one. "Is the other card in your possession, Ma'am?" Mr. Fraud enquired. "Well, yes, kinda, in a manner of speaking …" Good grief, why can life be so complicated before you have even poured your second cup of joe. Where did I see it last? I know it was nestled in that lovely cream-colored Coach pouch I like to take to games or places where I don't want to use up much space. I normally keep it in its matchy-matchy cream purse. Was it there? Of course not. I pull out all the bags I had used in recent weeks. Gosh what a lot of nothing one can accomplish some days. No, no and no. I go through my work bag – maybe it was nestling in there. No. How about the bag I use to transport things back and forth to work. Negative.

"When did you use it last?" husband asked, trying to be helpful. I ate up his helpfulness with my scowl.

"The other portion of your vacation rental is due today!" the cheery email came across. Ah, they need a card. No, not that card. I about slammed shut my computer, pulled up the covers over my head and canceled the day entirely. Somebody was messing with me, and it wasn't even Friday the 13th. "Is it too early for wine?" I enquired of our transaction coordinator. "Never!" came back her immediate response. I love that chick.

I finally put on some clothes, worked the ranch, washed my hair and put a little color on my face. Sometimes how you look can mirror how you feel, or make you change how you feel? Not really, but I thought I had better give it a go because the day was yet young and, so far, it had been super iffy on the accomplishment scale. As I was washing my foul start right out of my hair, it came to me. The blessed card was in my laptop case. Old smarty pants here had imagined that would be a safe spot to keep it, not thinking that she would immediately forget all about it. Ah, the card has been found. Yay me! Now to start ploughing through the phone calls I would have to make because someone thought they needed tickets to the New York ballet at my expense. How can that happen? It can and does much more often than it should, in my opinion.

Early afternoon and I had stopped going backwards in my quest to accomplish something, anything of positive note. A much-improved email zoomed through the ether. "Your book proof will be arriving on Tuesday!" My co-author and graphic designer in the UK would be receiving hers today. Today! How darn exciting is that! The story of our shared childhoods on the East Coast of England was just about ready for the open market and we felt like we had entirely birthed a very large baby over the course of the last 18 months or more.

"Oh, I have to make some color changes to the cover," she says all graphic-designery. Of course you do. It's not like we are going to make the Christmas rush with this tome, although mid-March is looking pretty good for a book signing in my hometown. My epic adventurer of a friend – my oldest friend in the world, no less, also co-author and graphic designer extraordinaire – is about to start her *Clipper Round the World* sailing race next month. Like a complete star, she is doing not one but two legs of the race, and those of us who prefer dry land can only stand back and be amazed at her bravery in heading out onto the ocean wave for a month to try and win a race. I take my non-sailing hat off to her and I shall be charting her progress like a pro. When she returns from Leg 1, we shall be inserting our book signing into the madness that will be her life, as she catches up with work and prepares to leave the UK for the US. Again. (Her husband is American. Every few years they have to move from one continent to another). Leg 2, she will be sailing from Seattle on her birthday, no less, and I shall be one of the 'Support Crew' (faker) in a blue t-shirt, waving a flag from the quay and no doubt bawling my eyes out like a complete pro, without ever stepping on a boat.

By the afternoon of this bad day, I was over the whole card thing, I was completely enthralled and excited by our new book and its possible launch in the next several days. I was anticipatory of our 2024 adventures in Seattle and a nice hotel already booked down near Pike Place and I felt super glad to be alive all over again. Now if I could just feel as chill about my oldest friend racing around the world on a boat, no less; things would be really good in my world.

(2023)

Bright Ideas

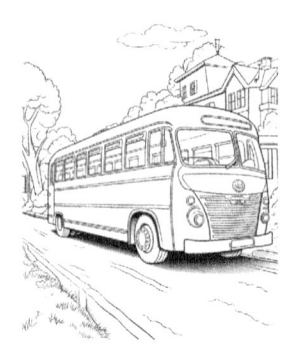

It was definitely my idea. Not my finest; but one I couldn't deny. There was going to be the National Association of REALTOR (trademark designation in capital letters NAR that we pay a great deal for!) meetings and exposition in San Francisco this year. The annual conference moves around the country, so it is quite the big deal when it lands in your neck of the woods. Meanwhile, our local Association was touting an Oktober Fest and the like. Why were we not going to be attending our NAR meetings, only 2 hours or so north or us? Enquiring minds – like my own – wanted to know.

I've been in real estate for a long time – well before I moved to the US. I used to work for my friend's bro-in-law in London when I was just a nip, showing properties and acting as if I knew what I was doing. It is one of those careers that gets inside your blood. Sometimes you love it and sometimes … well, you know. I still try to stay engaged and educated when I can. If you continue to do something as a job, you should do it as well as possible. And so, with my barky complaints, the bus trip to the NAR meetings in San Francisco was born.

I told my friend and colleague about it, and she was game, despite the early start. "It's good to stay educated," I persuaded her. "Learn about the new things in the industry, stay engaged." She was immediately sold. I picked her up at the crack of dawn. Mists swirled around the streets. It was dark and I hadn't had enough coffee. There is never enough coffee at that time of day.

Off we went with open minds, eager to learn. There were about 10 of us aboard a bus intended for 60 odd humans, most strange. So many had not thought this a valuable adventure; others flaked at the last minute – rather sad. Other people's time is seldom a valuable commodity, I thought, as we waited an extra 30 minutes for latecomers to the party who didn't show in the end. My friend and I had traveled a mere hour in dark and fog to be on-time for our bus ride. However, the extra coffee and pastries were much appreciated as we took off and soon arrived in the streets of San Fran as the people were awaking. The conference was already moving along when we entered the expansive halls (wrong place, first of all, and then across the street to the right place – such country bumpkins that we are), and we went into one of the expo halls to collect as many pens 'n' stuff as we could and see what we could learn. You forget about these large conferences. They basically want your money. They want you to pay for any additional knowledge you might infuse and so, it came to pass, that we only had access to the expo halls where they wanted to sell you stuff, not the educational forums where you could actually learn things. Not entirely true, but close.

By about 11am, we had collected all the pens and old Halloween candy that we could, and we were looking for coffee. I momentarily thought about standing in line to meet – randomly – Billie Jean King, famous tennis player – who must have got lost on the way to a senior tournament; we had no real clue why she would be at a real estate expo – but the line was long and I felt quite sorry for the lady, having to smile and hug lots of strangers in succession. We had our faces – also randomly – put onto cookies and took new photos for our business cards, lest they still be boasting the smiling, line-less images of yester-year, as some do. We ate a nice lunch near the conference halls and visited a few more booths. Finally, it was time to head south again and so we did. The bus driver was one of those *professional* drivers that needs a refresher course, if ever I saw one, and we were all feeling pretty queezy, as he lurched his way out of the city. Then we came to a halt, - not really, lurch lurch – and discovered that the freeway had been closed. Agh, things were going from bad to worse. I could feel my travel sickness affliction rearing its ugly head as it can do in such situations. Many others were feeling the same. Lurch lurch. "Get me a bag, please," I asked my colleague, and she did. It was a bit of an expo-porous type and dripped all over my jeans as I filled it. I was not happy. It reminded me of my boat trip from Athens to Crete when I was young. 12 hours on a boat, on a rolling sea and I was sick the entire time. Ever want to die, like really die? Yeah, be seasick for that long. Once I progressed onto plastic bags, my jeans and shoes were spared, but then the odor – oh the odor. It took us about an extra 1.5 hours to get home and I could not wait to get off that bus. My sea legs were so shaky I could barely walk. Then we drove home in the swirling fogs and arrived home late-late. "How was the conference, dear?" came the cheery voice of the husband who had, smartly, elected to stay home all day and was enjoying his television shows. "I'm headed to shower and bed," I croaked, pale as generic vanilla ice cream. "I feel like death."

And so it was that my bright idea to go to the National Association conference turned into a nightmare of epic proportions that I shall not repeat. Do not ask me to go on another bus, like ever. I won't go. I won't even volunteer to others that it might be a good idea. Some mistakes you will make only once in a lifetime. In my case, that is not entirely true, (see bus trip across the former Yugoslavia); but I won't do it again from where I'm standing right now. You cannot trust that the freeway will be open, and the driving skills of a so-called professional driver may just leave you speechless.

(2019)

Competition

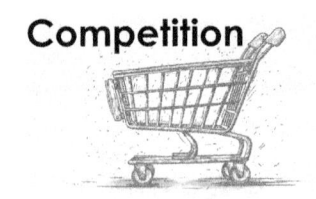

When I first moved to this little farm town, we had no proper grocery store, just corner markets. Actually, we boasted no larger stores at all! We had to travel to Greenfield to shop at Nob Hill or buy everything in Salinas before we commuted home. When our very own shopping center was under construction and a large household name grocery and drug store put into place, the smaller shopkeepers were not surprisingly alarmed; but look, they are mostly still here! They have developed their niche; they've learned that to survive, you have to diversify. Some carry nice fresh produce, others a decent meat counter, many some down-home friendly service you might not find in a larger establishment. Chain restaurants came into town, but look again, our small, local eateries are still here. Competition is good – it makes all of us better at what we do.

I was excited when I heard that Grocery Outlet was coming – finally, an increased choice in our grocery shopping options! Where there is little to no competition, a lackadaisical attitude can set in that does not promote very good customer service or quality products. At times in our larger grocery store, you could find yourself wishing you had gone to the corner market that time instead. Okay, so maybe the choices are not all there, but you could certainly make do with what was there, and you would be out of there in way less time. What price is our time? I also got tired of the large-name drug store and its long lines and excessive prices with empty shelves looking like no one could really care less. I moved my account to a local store where they know my name and can be informed and interested about my healthcare needs. You don't mind paying a bit extra for that.

And here we are. The new grocery store is open and there are nice extra choices to be found – not to mention different types of cheese and wine that we enjoy, also a wider selection of pet food and dog treats that we so appreciate. I believe there's room for both stores – I really do.

Not having found some of the things on my list at the new store, I went over to the old one. I was very disappointed. The shelves were pretty bare, loading carts were in the aisle, blocking your vision and accessibility, and there were not many people on the floor or working the tills. You would think that they would be on their best behavior, with their very best foot forward, now the new store is open and ready to steal their customers! With the other little towns passing by each day and easy on and off access for shopping, I think ultimately that both the stores will continue to do just fine.

And now they say that we will have a Dutch Coffee, Famous Footwear, Wing Stop, Panda Express and more in the same location! We are becoming quite the happening little place that was illustrated on the shirt and billboard years ago and laughed at by most, when, seriously, there was very little happening in Soledad. The powers that be are making it so that South County can keep their sales tax dollars more local, finally, and that is a win-win for all. Keep jobs and money and tax local – that will be helpful for all of us. And don't forget about the Tuesday specials at the movie theater in Soledad – that makes me so very happy! I love to go to the movies and appreciate it so much that they are here on my doorstep and making efforts to earn our business. With the Oscars showing on the television this weekend, I shall be scrutinizing the winners and seeing what I'd like to see in the coming weeks at my local theater on the big screen. Support local – it is so very important to keep communities intact!

For my part, during the foreclosure epidemic, all kinds of real estate entities moved into town and thought they would steal others' businesses. I remember being a little confused by how much business they thought was really here at the time. These wealth seekers came in, looked around, did a little business – not all good – and, mostly, left. There wasn't a darn thing any of us could do about it – competition is legal in the western world, and it is mostly a good thing. It keeps all of us on our toes.

Our company is still here in business where we were when Mary Poppins and her entourage floated into town and then rapidly left. And so are many other local businesses. When so-called competition arrives in town on the stagecoach, we just saddle up, tighten our boot strings and get better at what we do. It's a true story the world over.

So, I'm thrilled that we will now have more choices for our people in this town. I'm delighted that the other smaller towns nearby will likely stop by into our little town and spend their money here. I'm so happy that there will be jobs for people who want to work locally and occupations for our young people to earn a little cash and, in turn, help their families. This is the wonderful sign of a growing community that keeps pushing up like the crops in our fields on our luscious valley below. We are so lucky to live where we do and, increasingly, we don't need to go anywhere else to run our errands – buy our shoes and clothes, find some international cheeses, get some decent physiotherapy, or new tires, and go to the movies. I call that a great sign of progress in a small community and I want to commend all the folks who had a hand in this for a job very well done.

When I look back to when I bought a home here well over 22 years ago, this is an almost unrecognizable place –yet it remains totally recognizable and is still a nice place to live.

(2023)

Cowgirl on the country circuit

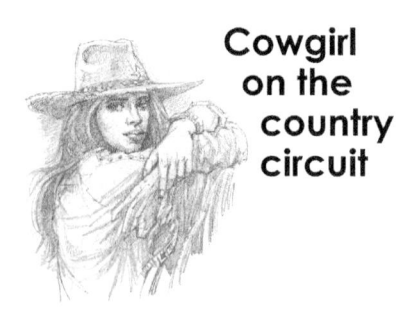

I've been on the concert circuit again the last couple of weeks. My poor husband sees me pulling out the cowboy hat and asks, wearily, "where is it this time?" He's not much of a concert goer these days, although – truth be told – he would have enjoyed Willie, but I didn't have an extra ticket for him! Ever since my daughter got me hooked on country music – yes, it's her fault of course – I have been on a crash course of emergency music education that ranges from the original roots of Willie Nelson – oh, be still my beating heart – to Blake Shelton, Kane Brown and more. And what a journey it has been. I used to diss country music. I love all kinds of music from classical to hard-ish; but I had always avoided that particular genre, even though I obviously lived in the country, rode horses, dressed like a cowgirl. You get the theme. In the end, there was an inevitability there. And then my daughter became the driver in my life when I go to visit her; and she is a country girl and plays country music without fail in her car! It was a little bit country by infusion.

My sister Rosie would ask me what tickets I wanted for my birthday or Christmas. She loved to buy the experience, in lieu of more stuff we don't need and I'm so glad she did. Over the years, she bought us hotel rooms, tickets to Adele, Coldplay, Rihanna, Jason and more. Now I look back and I'm so grateful for those fabulous times and many of them I experienced with my girl. And when Rosie took off for other planets, I took over her style of gift-giving. I have a feeling my daughter will take over the tradition down the road when I quit; she loves it so much.

So, on last week's agenda, was Tim McGraw at the California Rodeo Grounds – the kickoff to Rodeo week, if you like. We were all dressed and countried-up and ready for a good time. Sadly, since the Las Vegas horror, concerts have had to get super aggressive on the security front. You can't take in a regular bag, just an envelope-sized piece of ridiculousness that holds nothing, or a clear plastic bag that is just plain awkward. Once through the security, you have to get special wrist bands, that no one seemed to know where to find, so that you could buy a drink – maximum two – there are so many rules these days that, we understand, but could be fixed by some metal detectors and an ID registration when you buy the tickets? Anyway, serve to say, the enjoyment was a bit tempered by all the rigmarole and hurry up and wait for the audience who had paid well for the experience. The entertainer also seemed a little less than excited to be there. He didn't even greet the City of Salinas, the California Rodeo or introduce his band – I don't think so, at least. He certainly had no funny stories that I have come to expect from an entertainer – see Adele or Coldplay or Blake. Anyway, he did play some of the songs I liked, so it was fine.

The next week, I was headed South to the Cali Mid-State Fair to see my main man Blake Shelton – gosh, I do like that chap. Tall and grey and not too bothered by his fame and fortune, he really is a treat. Great stories, humor and songs and guitar and fiddle playing that can take you to other places you remember from the last time you saw him. There is something about live music that invades your soul and stays in your memory bank forever. The security there was much easier – body metal detectors and bag searches, thank you – and the whole experience a complete delight, it has to be said. Paso Robles also blessed us with some cooler temps than we expected in addition; so, the whole experience was beautifully memorable.

Thank you, Rosie, for giving us the unexpected gift of life experience so many years ago and reminding us of what is really important in life. At Blakey this week, we lifted our glasses to you and thanked you all over again. We know you were cheering from wherever you are these days in St Elsewhere – the other side of the curtain, just around the corner, down the street – and saying 'Go sister! That is so fab!" She loved it when I lived like I was dying – to coin a phrase – because aren't we all – and her tradition will live on in her absolutely fabulous memory to treat and spoil our generation, the next one and the one to follow.

This one is for you, my baby Bud.

Rosie Emma Alexandra Mason Arican died on July 25, 2018, after, what she would describe as, an amazingly full life, brimming over the top with wonderful experiences. She was 48-years old.

(2019)

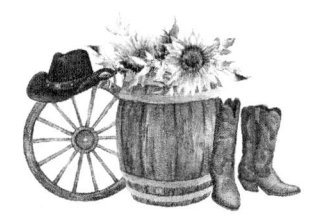

Delighted by the youth

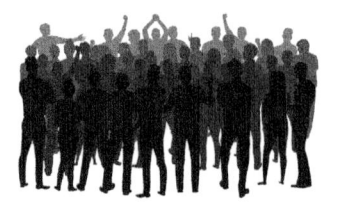

The South County Expo used to be a heck of an event here in town; but like all events, it takes people to host year after year and the people get tired. A couple of years ago, the Soledad Merchants Association elected to revitalize the event and host a showcase for local businesses, a forum for folks to share who they are and what they do. I always enjoy these get-togethers, a couple of hours of chatting to your neighbors in business and reminding yourself of what it is like to live and work in a small town. It's worth the effort to put yourself out there, for want of a better phrase, and be a part of your local community. Maria and Frank Corralejo spend an immense amount of their free time working on community projects to enhance life in this small town and it does not go unnoticed.

My business partner Letty and I had a booth each at the expo – one for our real estate business Legacy Real Estate group – and one for my bookshop LUNAbooks, (my book-writing hobby). With 5 titles to my name, it always makes me feel proud to set up my book shop wherever I go and realize that I accomplished my goal of being a published author, whether or not anyone actually buys and reads the books.

We were greeted at the expo by a group of young people in green shirts. They asked if they could help carry our stuff into the hall. This was a nice touch. They were members of a Workforce group that assist in the communities and get work ethics and experiences that will help them in future life. I thought that a marvelous idea. Another great idea was the entry fee being a few cans of unperishable food to benefit the Salvation Army. We can easily forget what tremendous work the Sally Army does for those in need – meals provided, food baskets handed out, shelter provided and so on. If you are in need, they will help you. Reminding people of the importance of their work was a lovely touch to a pre-thanksgiving event.

All of a sudden, I realized that several of the workforce students were standing in front of my booth. "What exactly is it that you do?" they asked me. A direct question from a young person struck me as interesting. I explained that I was a local columnist and author, also a REALTOR as my day job. "Oh, you have two jobs?" they enquired. "Well, no. I have a job and I have a hobby." I tried to explain to them that you do not always get to have the two things merge as one and they found that rather inspiring, it seemed. They wanted to know about each one of my books and what they were about. This was an on-the-spot interview I hadn't anticipated. I asked them if they read books and if they would like a book. To my surprise they all wanted a book. If they didn't have any cash on them, (maximum price for them $5) then I gave them books anyway. I was so delighted to have come across a group of young people who seemed as excited by books as me. Then they wanted the books autographed. "I can't believe I am standing in front of a real-life author!" exclaimed one. Had to giggle at that.

If you would have asked me about my expectations for the expo, I would have said that I would have chatted mildly with a couple of folks about the state of the real estate market. (Rates are still high, low inventory, blah blah.) A few people would have asked if the bookmarks and pens were free (yes) and I would maybe have sold a couple of my books, if I was lucky. Plus, the candy trays would have been emptied. I was literally blown away by this group of Workforce kids who were so personable and interested in the world. I know they will all do well. I commended their supervisor on what a lovely group of young people he brought along to our event. I really love to be pleasantly surprised in this life.

If you have a youngster in your life and you are not sure how to get them on a good path to life, I would urge you to check out the Workforce group and all their good works. I shall be keeping an eye out for them in the future.

"I've already got through 2 chapters," chirped one young man at the event, holding up one of my books. "It's so good!" If there was ever a reason to keep writing, this group gave me several.

Thank you, South County Expo and the Corralejo's for hosting another great event. I look forward to next year's and hope that my Workforce kids will be back and ready to read some more of my books.

What a wonderful time we had at our local expo. I went home that night with my heart very full of optimism and promise for the next generation.

While you are feasting around your dinner table this Thanksgiving, spare a thought for those you have food anxiety in their families and maybe send a few dollars to the Salvation Army folks who feed people year-round, not just during the holidays. It is a real and present need in our communities that we cannot ignore.

https://montereycountyworks.com

MCWDB-greencadre@co.monterey.ca.us (Green Cadre)
https://www.salvationarmyusa.org

(2023)

Making the time for tea

For the last few years, the first Saturday in December has been crowned the *Tea Party* fundraiser for the animal rescue. It's a nice, civilized way of getting people together and raising a few dollars for the vet bills. Joining with the Soledad Museum enabled us to have a decent downtown location to host the event – never mind the rain or shine – and meant that both groups could raise a little money together in the spirit of the season. This year we also added a baked potato fundraiser and though the Christmas parade itself was postponed by a week, that did not put a dampener on our parade, as it were.

In charity work there are few things that annoy me more than folks committing to help and then finding something else to do with their time. Fortunately for us, this was not a labor-intensive event this time, because we had a couple of very busy and dynamic elves – the Grisetti sisters that were – who made it their mission ever since the last tea party to search for china teacups and items for gift baskets as well as the baskets themselves; otherwise, we would have been in an awful mess. Mary Ann and Catherine painstakingly sought out, purchased, washed, dried and wrapped close to 100 china teacups and saucers over the last several months: no mean feat! The Museum folk and a few others took hours out of their day to bake and prep for the high tea, I cleaned out my tea pots, purchased milk and made sure the kettles were working for my part as Chief Tea Lady and made sure we had the auction sheets for the Silent Auction event.

Our student athletes can always be counted on to show up and work for us and they didn't disappoint us this time either. It is quite something to watch teenagers learning the art of pouring a decent cup of English tea. I always make sure they take a cup and saucer home as a souvenir of the occasion, and they seem to enjoy it! Surely not the toughest way to accumulate your school hours.

At the end of the afternoon, the volunteers were all pretty bushed and the tea goers full of tea and home-baked goods. There were several who thanked us for the nice occasion and noted that this was their chance to catch up with their friends in a nice, relaxed fashion. One lady added that, since she no longer drove, this was quite the highlight of her holiday season. That was touching. It's nice to host a quiet event where people take the time to sit down and talk to one another, sip a little tea and spend some money on worthy causes, especially during the holiday season. Two young men attended the tea party – I believe they were brothers. They told me it was their first time trying English tea and they were curious about it.

Another lady asked what sort of tea it was and where she could buy it. Some of the *young ladies* who attended have come every year and must have quite the tea service collection going on at their home. People enjoy it – pure and simple.

Every time I say I am retiring from working an event such as this, I am heartened by the smiles on the people's faces and pushed to say, 'well never say never …' It is lovely to have occasions that are more than about money – they are about people and human interaction hosted in a pleasant environment. I didn't hear a harsh word all afternoon and no one played games on their phones or checked social media.

Thanks to all who came and shared and donated to the event. Every slice of your contribution added to the completeness of the pie and, money or not, I'd like to say that it was a very successful day.

(2019)

Never too old

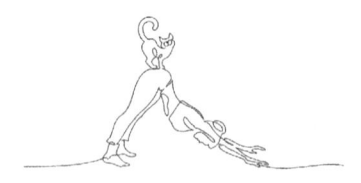

I first tried yoga about a month ago. I am not necessarily proud of that fact. Over the years, so many friends and family have counseled me to try it, give it a go, open up my mind to the possibilities. Even my mother – hardly an athlete of any kind – was a die-hard yogi for many years. I just never felt the pull. Until it came to me – obviously very late in life – that I might be able to use some of the stretching and breathing exercises at the very least.

I attended a class with my sister who is a relative newcomer to the *practice*– but, fair to be said, she will participate in anything that keeps her body moving. Though I was very clumsy and stiff, I enjoyed the session. Whether it was the conscious breathing or simply the peacefulness, I couldn't figure it out, but I came away wondering if I might need some more of that stuff to assist the body bits that are achy or creaking these days. My stupid knee injury has taught me way too much about the tedious timeline for successful healing when you are – ahem – a tad past middle age.

I returned home and husband was complaining about his stiff shoulder. "We should do yoga," I tell him. And then I see that he has already purchased a mat and blocks for his knees. What was going on here?

Our first yoga session was on *YouTube* with the beautiful lithe and supple Adrienne. She was so lovely and patient with her *Yoga for Seniors* calming voice intact. She made you feel as if it was okay if you couldn't get up off the floor very quickly or actually at all – a chair would suffice – as long as you kept breathing and working on your *practice*. (You learn a new language when you break into the yoga world.) But we felt we could do this – even us stiff old pensioners. There we were – down on the mat doing our cat poses, or *tabletops*, and it all felt pretty darn good and doable. We would finish after the 20-minutes or so with our muscles nice and warm and our halos shining. We both admitted to feeling more supple already after our first class and continued to repeat the same session several more times. Who knew there was such a wealth of coaching and training videos on YouTube? They are surely not making them for the money or the glory, but us oldies out there in tv land really appreciate all their hard work.

'You had a yoga trainer come to the house?' Our daughter was incredulous. 'Na, just Adrienne.' I replied cryptically. 'A chick from YouTube'. 'Omg, dad is really doing yoga?' I could sense her curiosity had been piqued. Our son too. 'Dad is doing YOGA???' The text came over from the depths of Sacramento. Increasingly, I think more men are appreciating the benefits that yoga can give them and it's quite a unisex practice; though husband has never been one to jump right in and participate in any kind of sport. This has been rather a nice surprise for all.

This weekend would have been my mother's 90th birthday and I wonder what she would have made of all this yoga practice going on at Solace. She would likely have sniffed and said it was about time I absorbed all its many benefits, before advising me to not immediately try and stand on my head or I would break my neck.

It feels good to try new things. Whether or not, you can get up from the floor once down there and then the bursts of giggles mean that you definitely cannot rise from the mat anytime soon; or the dogs decide to try and do some *downward dog* with you and hang very close to you on the mat, you must not be distracted. The early morning breezes stream in through the screen door and the calming mists over the Salinas River bring to mind all the opportunities of the new day ahead. It's a good way to start the day, even if you really suck at the *practice*.

I don't think I've ever paid so much attention to breathing in my entire life; but Adrienne tells you to listen to your body and focus on your consistent inhaling and exhaling and that feels like a simply good thing to do. I've observed that I hold my breath when I get tense and I wonder if I have always done that. It can't be good for one, and I shall endeavor in the future to be more like Adrienne. She's a solid breather.

I don't know if we will ever graduate to Adrienne Part 2, or perhaps a You Tube class for the Seniors who now know how to do a little yoga, but I'm glad we found it, however late in life, and however appalling we are at the practice. I'm enjoying the release of tension and the exchange of oxygen, even if some of my twists and turns and stretches could be a little more impressive in scope and style. As Adrienne would say, *the intent and the integrity* are there.

I'm happy to learn yoga and whatever she can teach me about improving my mobility and easing up my creaky bits for the rest of my life to come. I may not be able to run a marathon anymore – truthfully never could. I may struggle sometimes to walk my dogs as much as they would like and I no longer ride horses, but guess what, I can do yoga, whatever that means. I can try something new that will likely benefit my body and how lucky am I to have the opportunity! Embrace the new gifts that come along in life and let go of the youthful activities you can no longer enjoy. Inhale and exhale, it can be as simple as that. Give it a try.

Take kindly the counsel of the years, gracefully surrendering the things of youth –

Desiderata

(2023)

The Lost Week

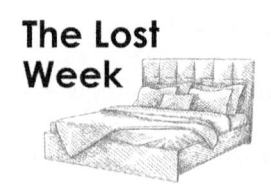

"Sick in bed, dude." The message came over from my son who had spent a couple of days with us the previous week. "Ugh," I respond. "I have a sore throat."

"Yes, dude, that's how it starts."

Some weeks just happen to you, when you are making other plans. This was not good. I had animals to take care of, work to do, houses to close. I couldn't be sick; just could not. It would pass me by and latch onto others more deserving, for sure. I hadn't been sick for a very long time. I'd ignore it and it would go away. Self-employed people don't get sick pay, so they cannot be sick, right?

Tuesday, I felt dreadful, just dreadful. I could feel the anvil of doom hanging over my head. I was about to get slammed. I quickly accomplished everything that absolutely had to be done at my desk, hacking and spluttering the while. I couldn't breathe and my head was pounding. We won't even talk about the other end.

There's nothing quite as divine as the cool white sheets of your own bed when you're feeling really lousy – even during the daytime. And there she was, waiting for me. The breeze flowed through the screens, the birds were singing, it was bright daylight outside, and I was under the covers. If I don't awaken from an afternoon nap before 8pm, I know there's something very wrong with me. My dogs were all lying around my sick bed, dealing with the boringness of their afternoon and willing me to feel better, so we could go outside and play ball, as usual. This was not the Mama they knew and loved. Must be something to do with that missing white horse that everyone kept talking about. They couldn't figure it out.

Tomorrow I would feel better. Nope. "Yeah, there's a nasty virus going around," she said, helpfully. "Lasts for weeks!" Weeks? I don't have days, let alone weeks. Still felt terrible. Tried to get moving, tried to stop sniveling and hacking, didn't work. "Mono, dude." The message came across from my son. "That is not even remotely funny!" I spit back. (When you are under the weather, you have no sense of humor, by the way!) "I'm still sick, dude," he added as an after-thought. What was this, the flu? (Yes, I had had the shot) ... one of those super bugs that were slaying people the world over? (Us sickies can get pretty melodramatic in addition!) I felt insulted by the affliction.

The next day I would wake up with a clear head and not need to spend the entire day in bed. I knew it; just knew it. Didn't happen. I found myself dragging my feet up and down the corridors of my house like dead-woman walking. "Better dear?" the husband broaches, cheerfully and hopefully. "Nope.." I say deadpan and shuffle my way back down the corridor to my bed. There's nothing worse in the world than a sick woman; except for, possibly, a sick man.

Last week is a fug I tell you and also a fog, if you're not sure what a fug is. I mean it's all a bit of a blur, meshed up with cold and cough medicines and sleep aids that, by the way, do not assist with the memory. Boxes of tissues and, also, the lovely used kind litter the house and fall out of every sleeve and pocket, as I endeavor to get myself showered and dressed and back to work. Several days down the road, I have still lost the use of my left nostril and there's a scaly red circle around my mouth and up to my nose and over my inflamed nostrils, but, at this point, I think I will, ultimately, survive this Mega-Super-Virus of 2019 and I will, eventually, rediscover my sense of humor, likely located somewhere around the corner from the cold and cough aisle at the pharmacy, where, I believe, I am now, not only, just inspiring armlengths worth of *Buy More Of Me Cold and Cough Medicine* Coupons, but also the possibility of an invite to be an investor in all of their companies.

This is a true story. I am not asking for your sympathy for my lost week, the wasted days of my life, the anguish of my bored-to-death puppies and the apparent suffering of my husband. No, I'm just giving you a warning that, if you wake up with a sore throat and it's not diagnosed as mono, it's likely the super virus plague of 2019 knocking at your door and – heads up – you'd better take the rest of the week, or year, off.

(2019)

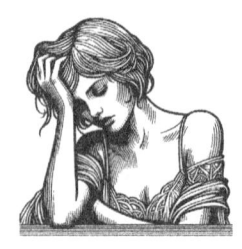

The Waiting

The Waiting is the worst. I don't think there is anyone who would challenge me on that. I get flashbacks to my own cancer diagnosis from over 10 years ago. One test slowly crawled to another and you are in the waiting room of your life, imagining that the disease will have spread over your entire body before you have even got to the stage of pre-op. I was about 6-8 weeks from diagnosis to surgery and I very nearly lost my mind. I'm sure we are not alone in our current frustrating situation, nor our now compounding stack of medical bills that promises to grow exponentially over the coming days. I haven't been in this situation for a while and, I'm remembering now, it's a frightening and lonely place to be. Fresh on receipt of a near $8K – our cost after insurance – emergency visit with husband who is not eligible for unemployment nor disability, being one of the nation's self-employed; we are swiftly reminded of the need for the rainy-day fund, the back-up plan. The blank-blank can and does happen in the blink of an eye.

In my case, going back the decade or so, we were lucky we had things to sell to be able to manage this enormous surprise that hit us like a freight train with my diagnosis and my multi-hospitalizations thereafter. We sold both of our investment properties, our beautiful VW cherry classic '56 Bug and our super classic '63 VW split window bus. We had nothing more to sell but our house after that and we were still in debt with medical bills for many years after. Fortunately, and thanks to family generosity, we were able to keep our beloved roof over our heads. But honestly, an unfortunate encounter with illness can push you to that financial cliff over which you could lose absolutely everything – because you get sick? I think there is something wrong with a system that finds that acceptable.

We pay insurance to a company. We have a choice of plan, but no choice of company. Shouldn't there be a selection of companies, some competition in the health insurance marketplace? Why isn't there any competition? Are the health insurance lobbyists for that particular carrier so deeply in the pockets of who knows who, that no one questions how this is an equitable situation for the insurance buying public.

Years ago, when I worked for a Fortune-500 company and was blessed with the most amazing insurance package I never appreciated, I paid my small contribution to the insurance and received superb care. The birth of my child, for instance, a c-section with complications, only cost me $500 and I do believe that to be a little low from where I'm currently standing; but I think things have got sorely out of wack in our current situation. Where's the competition? Where's the gate keeper for these preposterous bills that regular people can never pay?

Civilized countries across the world manage a health-insurance-for-all situation. Why can't we? The folks who can pay some should pay some. I don't think anyone would argue about that. But, United States style, being forced into a corner when somebody has a heart problem that requires multiple tests and likely procedures, with unaffordable medical bills the result? I see now how people lose everything through medical misfortune. We nearly did 10 plus years ago, and we still might this time around. We don't have anything much left to sell, but isn't that a sad reflection on honest working folk who encounter hard times? We are not young; we have no more investment properties or classic cars to sell. We are just working people who are down on our luck and this misadventure could break us all over again.

Meanwhile, it is fortunate that my husband seldom reads my columns, because he would flip out if he thought that $8K was our contribution towards his first of many doc visits this past month or so. I can't tell him because he is already riddled with anxiety at the waiting that is required within the health system, at his own feelings of inadequacy that he has no money coming in or ability to do anything about that and I am, meanwhile, trying to cover all bases while we figure out what is wrong. The referral from one doc leads to the waiting for another doc. "Oh he is booked for another month," she says. Husband's response – "I might be dead by then. Is there no one else we can see?" "Oh yeah, you can see so and so in 3 weeks." What? You try to advocate for your own care, only to be shot down, when there is no one available to see what they deem to be your non-emergency situation; and yet your own clock is ticking and your mortality dangling by a thread.

I know lots of clever people have tussled with this issue over the years. We, as one of the world's super-powers, should surely be able to figure out a better plan than the one we currently have. Pay your health insurance bill and all will be well, as long as you are; because when you are not, there is a tsunami of horror awaiting you in the mailbox as well as in your imagination, not to mention your financial situation. You are waiting, you are waiting some more; and you feel that no one really cares except for you and your loved ones. "Yeah, we have to get that approved through your insurance!" What? My life is on the line. "Yeah, we'll see if the insurance covers that." I flash back again to arguing with the insurance over the double mastectomy I was demanding, when they just wanted to approve a lumpectomy. The 3rd female in my family to be diagnosed with breast cancer and they didn't want to give me the operation I needed. I will never forget that. My old dad even offered to pay for the double mastectomy out of his own pocket.

So, what's the solution for all the smarty pants to figure out? We definitely need some competition in the health insurance arena – I think that goes without saying. Health care costs need to be reviewed and addressed. (Don't give me a huge bill without itemizing every darn cost that you put down there!) Working people have no issue paying towards their care; but surely an equitable playing field would be that you contribute towards health care, but it doesn't entirely take your whole life down the tubes? Friends of mine in Europe are aghast when I tell them about our health care costs – it literally blows their mind. Their system is not perfect – it certainly is oversubscribed – but neither is ours. I wonder when this topic might become a priority; I'm hoping in my lifetime to see a workable solution. In the meantime, I don't have the means to pay the $8K, so I shall no doubt be collecting some bad credit and increased debt, while I strive to heal my husband within this broken, inequitable system.

(2020)

SECTION 5

Me & It

Introduction to - Me & It*

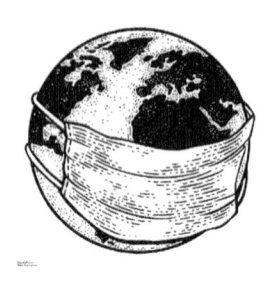

If we really think that 2020 needs any introduction at all. As my granddaughter Madison Rose aptly named it, *that stupid coronavirus**. And what a year that was! The new language that was learned and behaviors adopted. From N95 masks to distance learning to global runs on toilet paper and refrigerated trailers in hospital parking lots; it was the makings of a very bad movie, but, sadly, it became our lives, our new normal. We didn't want it to be our normal, we wanted to get our old lives back and take back our lost freedoms. When we were not being impatient humans, there were some lovely views to be had along the way of clear skies, people growing their own veggies and baking their own bread, neighbors keeping an eye on one another, life slowing down, quiet streets – nearly like a reset of the entire world.

We are an impatient species, humans. We cannot stand darkness that is imposed upon us – we cannot tolerate lockdowns or being told where we can and cannot go, what face coverings we must wear on our noses and mouths, or any other kind of restriction to our free lives that we resent holding back on. 'Bring on 2021! Good riddance to 2020… Cannot wait for this awful year to be over' ….

2020 was quite the year, wasn't it. It was a year that went on and on and became 2 years in all actuality. The year 'plus' when, unimaginably, the world shut down, planes didn't fly, trips didn't happen, schools closed. Everyone was socially distanced and awkward and, horrifically, too many people died of this awful virus.

A new language evolved during lockdown. Pandemic, bubbles, essential workers, staycations, social-distancing, PPE, Zoom, distance-learning, N95's and more. Our essential workers – our nurses, fire, police, (even notaries, ha!) found themselves out there in empty streets, all masked up, (some in space suits) with latex gloves a must have, lots of disinfectant wipes and a new mask for every situation.

There were crazy runs on grocery stores the world over that went in phases. Initially it was for the masks, disinfectant wipes, gloves, hand sanitizer, paper towels and toilet paper, for crying out loud. I remember signs in the store advising that there was a 2-roll ration per household. Refrigerated trucks parked outside of New York hospitals was a memory that will never fade. These were some crazy, frightening times. The days and months without a vaccination frankly terrified most of us and separated many, as the vaccine debate became a political one that continues to divide our nation.

But then there were, thankfully, some bright sparks during darker days. With no airplanes flying or folks only traveling for a permitted hour outside their own homes, dolphins and swans were to be seen along the canals of Venice. Folks would open up the windows to their homes at designated times each day and cheer, all over the world, singing thank yous out into the fresh air to the essential workers who were putting their lives on the line every second they were on the floors of hospitals the world over, trying to save the lives of others. My daughter was one of those essential workers and I had to try and not think about the risks she was taking with her young life in the service of others. The photo she sent me of her small self, wrapped up in a space suit at work is one that made a mother's heart super anxious at the time, but also immensely proud.

Many of us ran, not walked, to the pharmacies the world over, once we were eligible for the first vaccine and followed through with all the others we were allowed to have. I remember my important little white CDC card I had to carry, showing the dates of my immunizations and which brand I had (Moderna). It became a part of my passport to the world, once I was able to travel again, the latter part of 2021.

And we were so impatient for the year to be over, as if the stupid coronavirus* would simply stop at the end of the year, ha! As if a new year would mean a re-set of all we had dealt with for 9 months of that year. We had some learning to do and it was not pretty. We had to learn that hope was not canceled. The day would come when we would not be subject to lock down and all things imprisoning in human perception. We had to learn that when the world locks down it will take a long time to open back up and that requires patience. We had to learn the new rules of traveling around the world. We had to learn a bunch of difficult lessons that did not sit well with the impatient public and our habits of being free to do whatever we please.

But I think we will all agree that, when the world edged back to some kind of normality, we were a bit older and wiser. We had stopped taking our freedoms for granted and we were all a bit humbled.

(*Courtesy of Madison Rose Jensen, aged 5, who had to do distance learning for over a year, another new piece of 2020 terminology. She lost her whole kindergarten year to that *Stupid Coronavirus*, and some say the young suffered more than the rest of us through that very challenging time.)

Thoughts about that? I'd love to hear.
lucymasonjensen@gmail.com

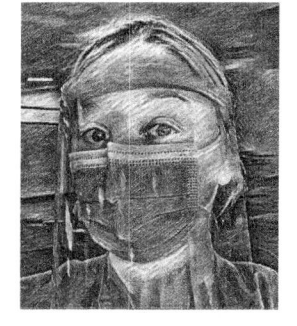

A week of firsts

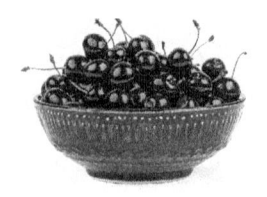

I've been digging rather deeply recently to try and find the good stuff in the world. I'm sure I'm not the only person to say that life is currently pretty tough. Coupled with my husband's illness and our financial stress, the wide-open spaces of the unknown this year in all capacities; and you got yourself a big old stress fest, that never seems to leave you even in sleep. I toss and turn, blaming the border collie on my feet for my white nights and wondering at the disturbing dream set in which I seem to continually be the main action figure. The moon smiles brightly in the window over my head, as if to say 'yes I know you are troubled. Have some more light to keep you awake.'

But there are always others with more troubles than your own and the pulse of America was beating hard in recent days with sadness, injustice, civil unrest and uprisings to add to this strange of strangest of years. I was concerned when I heard that 2000 people were going to be bussed into our small town for a *Black Lives Matter* march. There's nothing remotely wrong with people protesting; it's an important feature of our democracy. However, the looting and destruction in so many other places gave us considered cause for concern. Buildings started to board up their windows, folks closed their businesses and gave the employees the day off. I needed to work; so, I thought it best to go downtown and guard my plate-glass windowed store front and hope to be pleasantly surprised. I really was. The march came along in all shapes and colors with signs and doggies a part of it all. There was a respectful police presence and no unruly behaviors of any kind. It was actually quite moving to see the young people find their voices and show up for a cause they believed in. Here's hoping they keep showing up like that. With the November ballot box just around the corner, it's past time that everyone got up out of their chairs and became involved for the greater good.

This was the first week I ever took a knee in my life, and I did so at the march in my small town. I am a huge patriot, and this had nothing to do with not respecting our country and our flag; but supporting the rights of other human beings whose blood is the same color as mine will always be a priority for me. It felt like the right thing to do. A friend participant of the march told me that it brought tears to her eyes, seeing me by myself on the sidewalk on one knee, as the march went peacefully by.

This was also the week that I got my first Covid test. Listening to our governor talk about the importance of getting tested for the statistics and the continued re-opening of our State geared me up to go and get it done. Super easy. Google Greenfield, CA Covid testing, (located at the Greenfield library). Fill out a short questionnaire and choose your testing time. I was in and out in about 5 minutes. I felt almost as if I had done my civic duty and I urge others to do the same. There are so many variants to this unknown beast of a pandemic that we all need to give the powers that be whatever information might be useful to them, as we navigate these uncharted waters.

One good thing I will say about this very peculiar week was the opulence of our cherry crop at Solace. I have never seen such robust, sweet, dark beauties. We picked a whole load for cherry jam, and we ate a whole load more. Husband made a delicious spicy version, and we still have our trees swaying with their bounty. Even our peckish birds cannot keep up! On the tail of our *Covid Cherries,* we have a whole tree-load of *Pandemic Plums* ready to give us more bounty.

With all the chaos in the world, try to focus on the good stuff where you can and show up for rightful and constructive protest, whenever possible.

(2020)

Always look on the bright side

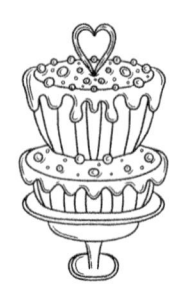

Easier said than done, I know. These have been some unprecedented months in the life of a year – and we haven't even made it to 6 of the blessed things yet!

I recently found myself popping into the local dollar store. I needed a birthday card, simple enough. But wait! I found myself actually picking up a basket and cruising the aisles for life's essentials. Who does that in a dollar store? I've obviously missed the art of browsing; I hadn't realized how therapeutic it is to just lose yourself in a retail environment and zone out mind and body. I exited the dollar emporium with quite a lot more than a greeting card I can tell you! I don't want to do curb side retail, I want to go inside and see what the styles and colors are, I want to look at the shoes on sale and browse the swim aisle for a new bathing suit to be worn on vacation in the latter part of the year. We can only hope. Hark! It's an airplane trail! Wait, there is more than one. I've missed those things! What is happening? Is the world opening up? Gosh your mind can go into a strange tailspin after 8 weeks of lockdown.

With feral feet peeking out of my flip flops, daring the world to say one word about closed nail salons, I scrape the last of the gnarly gel polish off my stubby thumb and wonder if it's time to teach myself how to pretty up the darn things. My hair is a nest of whirling grey-blonde wisp with split ends flying in the wind and I do realize that, during a Zoom meeting the like of which I had never heard of before March, it's quite fun to not have to wear any pants.

People I know are worrying about the end of lockdown and how they will feel when they are forced out again into the world. "I cried for the first 2 weeks," one said. "Now I'd like it to stay this way forever in my safe house with my puppies and my beloved. I can work perfectly well in my jim-jams from home. Don't make me go back!" She positively wailed. Another remarked how she was a social butterfly and just wanted to be able to go out to lunch with a friend, without having to mask up, go and stand 6 feet apart, buy the take-out to take home, heat it up, do the dishes. That is not a fun outing, nor a relaxing way to socialize with food.

I'm becoming my mother. I've realized this during lockdown. Rather than read about CV, how many deaths, how many sick, how far away is a vaccine, I find myself running away from all serious news, just as she did. I casually flick through all that muck, plus the obituaries of course, on my online device and delve into the new books to be bought, holidays to be taken, meals to be made amidst all the lifestyle and literary pages. My book stack has already grown a sister and is spilling all over the place. I keep finding more books I must buy. And don't even go there with the kindle thing! Can't do it. Not the same at all.

My friend, over the course of 8 short weeks, has become a baker and is bemoaning the lack of flour to be purchased. Flour, really? We have gone from toilet paper hoarding to paper towel and now flour shortages? Another friend of mine noted that she had become completely round during lockdown. She had found so many delicious things to bake like banana bread, chocolate biscuit cake and apple crumble (with custard) that she couldn't imagine what she was going to do when she had to actually leave the house and go to work again – paid – and not just search the online stores for flour and bake at will in her lovely country kitchen. Oh, and the gardening trend. Everyone is gardening these days. Even those with the off-green fingers are having a go, and, surprisingly, yours truly, a total non-gardener, could be seen to be doing a little therapeutic weeding on occasion, grabbing hold of those viciously persistent lil grassy monsters and enjoying ripping out their roots. (I miss my therapist, can you tell?)

Yes, in 2 short-long months, the world has gone completely bonkers and none of us know where we will be going from here. It's the biggest ol' muddle that most of us have seen in our lifetimes. So ….what to do when we are not baking or gardening, or buying more books? We can chat to our friends – on Zoom, Facetime or any other which way. That doesn't require a mask. We can dream about holidays in our newly purchased bathing suits, one day, and cruising along retail aisles that are not at the dollar or grocery store. We can even imagine, somewhere along the cliff edge of stage 5 lockdown, enjoying a nice meal with friends at a restaurant.

There are many things beyond our control during these strange days. Within our control is that we can strive to be cheery and look on the bright side of life. We are still here; still mostly smiling…. And sometimes even making ourselves laugh out loud.

(2020)

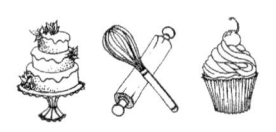

Covid Year 2

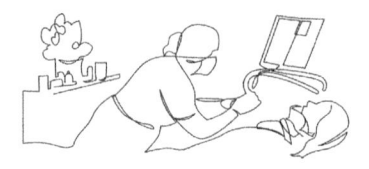

They said it would all be gone by now; it would have just been blown away like an errant feather – a dark memory from the archives of 2020. The last Christmas holidays, that should have been spent in my hometown on the English East Coast, now but a memory of all things lost and canceled by Covid during that dastardly year past. But here we are in the second year of restrictions, also known in some regions as *Panda* (a sweet name for pandemic), with intensive care units still taking over hospital gift shops and refrigerated trailers a lingering memory from last summer and continuing to occupy real estate in the parking lots of law enforcement the country over.

I was chatting to my friend in England and was relieved to hear that all the elderlies in her family have now been vaccinated. There is a tier system in place over there of summoning people for their turn, and stadiums and pharmacies are lined up to do their part in the coming days. We hope for that here. In the meantime, my daughter is a front-line medical worker and has not even received her first vaccine. My husband is vulnerable health-wise without a shot in sight and I shall be somewhere at the end of the line right before the teenagers. I'm not complaining, but someone in authority did tell us that Covid would just disappear a long time ago and that could not be further from the truth.

We are used to being free to make plans and enjoy times together. We are not a solitary breed, accustomed to staying in our houses and only dealing with folk in our bubble. Some of us are very used to traveling freely across the world and planning an entire year of adventures right at the beginning of each year. My friends and I are incessantly slotting in the next trip and marking calendars. My finger is always ready to book the next flight, indulge in hotel perusing and sights to see, places to go. It has seldom been enough for me to just stay in one place and be happy with my lot. I'm a gypsy at heart; probably always will be; likely how I ended up here, a long way from home.

But year two of Covid, with no end in sight, has forced me to be happier with my lot; to not plan every single thing. I am at the will of the scientists and the clever medical folks – also the vaccine planners – who will devise the correct plan for our State and my family in due course. They told us it would be easy; it's not. It was my baby sister's 51st birthday, (forever 48). I had planned a trip to a special beach in her honor, a place where I could also chat to my Mum and visit with the cormorants and pelicans – and occasionally the odd seal, otter or whale. I had the whole day aligned, even down to my favorite dish at my favorite restaurant after my beach walk. It was all going along swimmingly, that is until I forgot to check the tides and the King Tide explosion on this particular shoreline meant that there was little to no beach to walk upon and hardly a stick of driftwood to collect. I made my solitary pilgrimage along the ravaged sand, enjoying the shrieks of children playing in the surf and people picnicking on the sand. My favorite dish at my favorite place was not to be had. They had obviously got tired of the opening-closing-half-opening of the last 10 months and decided to heck with it, we'll just take a vacation and wait until restaurants can behave like restaurants again. We were starving and found a Thai restaurant open for take-out. That would have to do. Shop local and all. We picnicked in/out of the truck, and it was decent. I like a little bit of noodles with some seafood. Nowhere near the divine salivation of my favorite crab enchiladas, but there you go again with the Covid-disappoint factor, ever present in our regular lives and likely to remain so for a while.

My husband's aunt Marvel died in her sleep. We are all a bit of a flutter, because she had wanted to be buried with her husband George in Watsonville. She passed in Los Angeles and how the heck were we going to give her a proper send-off? How can you gather during Covid and do the normal respectful nods to a life well-lived when no one is allowed to gather and grieve and hug? I had heard that a gathering of 5 at a funeral is all you can do. Hers was a family of many more than that. Generations of beloveds of that funny little lady who would want to say their farewells. Maybe we will have to have a lottery of who gets to go, or we just Zoom and no one gets to go? I haven't the faintest idea.

One of my favorite transatlantic airlines just sent me an email that they would no longer be doing the long-haul flights, San Francisco to London. They owed me a flight from the one they canceled last May. That may be going the way of all the lost plans and broken dreams from 2020, now spilling over into 2021. The sad fall-out of one business after another, unable to survive in year two of this Crazy-Corona world. But they said it would all have gone away by now; business would be booming again and everything back better than ever. I think they lied. My father, on the Isle of Man, told me that they are back on lock-down again. They had a delightful 6 months of Covid-free living from summer to winter, but then the blessed virus showed up again on their island to remind everyone that moving freely is not free and it comes at quite a price these days. Dad is 91 and still has no idea when he will be receiving his vaccine. I think the world is in for a bit of a rollercoaster ride, before anything really improves on our planet and life post-Covid can resemble anything close to life before we even knew what a *Covid-Panda* was.

It's a bugger's muddle, as Granny would say. This *Panda* will teach us a few things about a few things, that is a for sure. Let's hope by year 3, the promises of the high-level people will come to fruition and we, the small people, can embrace our freedoms once more, as we are all desperate to do.

(2021)

Glass half full

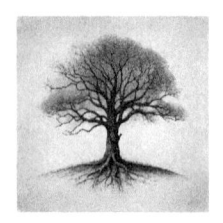

With the changing of the times and the lessening of the daylight, I must annually go on self-watch alert. There is something about darkness during the daytime that makes me – well – dark. I can get the gloomies very easily when the clocks fall back and, this year, I think it might be easier than most to tumble down the dark hole and lose myself for a few days, where I might find many others from the world. Except that that is not helpful for the universe, especially when I currently hold the dubious position of cheerleading nurse in the household, encouraging our resident patient to see the glass half full, even when he feels as if his recovery is too slow – one step forwards – two backwards – and is frustrated that he can't just jump in his truck and go off to work like a regular person.

We are an impatient species, humans. We cannot stand darkness that is imposed upon us – we cannot tolerate lockdowns or being told where we can and cannot go, what face coverings we must wear on our noses and mouths, or any other kind of restriction to our free lives that we resent holding back on. 'Bring on 2021! Good riddance to 2020… Cannot wait for this awful year to be over…' Many are wishing away their lives in some unrealistic expectation that January 1 of the New Year will herald the dawn of a new beginning, where big bad Covid is just a crummy memory and we will all start booking flights for our holidays for next year that just has to make up for this one. I don't see it, I'm afraid.

For now, I'm not booking anything for next year. And by that statement, I don't mean to be a Debbie Downer. Having canceled more holidays and flights that I dare to describe, because I refused to believe that a wretched virus could and would shut down all my 2020 plans, I am staying at home and biding my time. Those of you who know me will know that I don't say that lightly. I love to travel, live to travel! But no. We must listen to the medical expects; learn patience and wait for the vaccine, listen for the testing improvements and do our best to look on the bright side. Many of us have food in our cupboards and some source of income. We are the lucky ones. Can we help others less fortunate? We have health insurance, lest we need a major heart operation. Our human families are surviving, and our fur families don't have a clue – they just love it that we are home more these days. We are the lucky ones. And there are many out there who cannot say that. We must empower ourselves to be the cheerleaders in our circle of influence where we can. I try to do my part by sharing fabulous photos of my home and beasts and contributing to the cheer that way. People tell me that it helps. I aim to be grateful for my lot by feeding the wild birds, the hummingbirds, all the critters. I leave water out for the wild animals that might pass by in the night and need a place to lap and refresh. It's my way of encouraging the universe to look on the bright side too.

Fall has her own beauty, she really does. Some of the best sunset skies can be seen in the fall. The leaves are falling in divine cascades of color and the vines are hanging heavy with old fruit that feeds the wild animals and contributes to the economy of the valley. Fall is time for recollection of a year nearly done, for gathering thoughts and gifts. It's past time to clean out a cupboard and give to the needy. Could you buy an extra turkey for a family this Thanksgiving, or host a needy child with a slice of Christmas cheer?

Sometimes the daily burdens of our existence can weigh heavily – working, caregiving, managing – and we look only inwardly; especially when the afternoons are darkening too quickly and there is a nip in the air that pushes us to put away the summer whites and dig out the thick darks of winter. It's all part of the cycle that we must accept. Just like the cycle of a virus that crushes local economies and the lives and plans of many, the cycles rotate, and it will not be like this forever; just as winter annually blends into spring and spring to summer.

In the last portion of this difficult year, I am putting myself on a time-out to gather myself and find the gratitude in all I do have and not the other. As we move towards Thanksgiving and, likely, a quiet festive table this year, I hope to find there a peacefulness of quiet acceptance. With the darker days, maybe I can read more books and write more stories. Perhaps that cupboard will finally get cleaned out and I will package up goods for those who need things more than I do.

Hoping that you and yours can find your own slice of peace and acceptance too. Let's cool the rage and the divisiveness and remember the first Thanksgiving. Let's share what we have and be mindful of the less fortunate, as good people in good communities do. That can only serve to provide the sort of cheer I think we all need this year. Be sure, I shall be working on mine.

(2020)

Health and sickness during corona

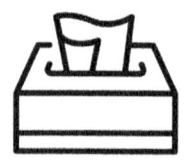

During your wedding vows – in less than good health and in slightly better health and all that jazz, you are so caught up in the romanticism of the prospect of – hopefully – being together forever, you don't really think about the sickness part of the vow. You just hope you will both stay healthy and go with that. And yeah, the older you get, the more that is not realistic. The medications and the syndromes and the sickness can become ever present in your world. They don't tell you about that part.

Me: "Did you take your medications?"
Him: "What?"
Me: "DID YOU TAKE YOUR MEDICATIONS?"
(Shouting and trying to use proper lip synch at the same time.)
Him: "Yeah!"
Me: "Did you take them with food?"
Him: "What?" (By now irritated … he's watching one of his many shows on television with the volume up …)
Me: (Shouting above the tv volume ….) "DID YOU …?" You get the picture. None of this is romantic and none of this is what you are imagining, as you make your vows to one another and look forward to years of wedded – and, you hope, healthy – bliss.

Move stage about 22 years forward in this house and the old man, (I use that term affectionately), has a bad ticker, a problem heart, heart disease if you like. There is really no good way to couch his condition in a romantic way. In March, he started to feel dizzy. I thought he was dehydrated, I thought he may possibly be pre-diabetic. (Don't ever Google symptoms. If you are not a doctor, stay away from any determination of condition! Lesson learned!) I thought he might have some type of digestion issue, since he always ate, near flat, in his stretched-out recliner, watching his shows. Nope, none of the above. His arrhythmia – that he was born with – could not even be blamed for the various cardiac issues, the like of which took the best part of 5-6 months to work through.

You start with the regular doc. Then the referral to the neurologist. No, he doesn't have a brain tumor, check. Then a cardiologist, actually two. They did a good clean-out of his arteries. Check. Problem not fixed. Then onto another cardiologist for a pre-ablation determination. Yup, need that. Back to the other. On to the other. All kinds of tests through all these procedures. Wait for insurance approvals. More waiting. And all of this during COVID, when the doctors don't want to see anyone in person, and they are really backed up with all the patients they haven't seen in ions. What a challenge this has been!

The day of his first ablation arrived … (top of the heart). During the times of Covid, you get to drop them at the hospital like they are catching an airport bus and then leave. That is a very strange feeling. No stressing out in the waiting room with other nervous families. No eating limp-ass food in the cafeteria with other peeps in the dark zone of their lives. Nope. You pull up at a place where it seems everyone is catching an Uber to or from a concert. You drop off your patient and you leave. The rest of the day is dark zone itself. I thought I was going to stress-clean, but I couldn't even do that. Nurse Jackie called from the hospital a few hours later and told me he was coming around and would be able to come home later. And then, when he was more or less awake, he texted that he might be able to and then he said he wasn't and then he was. The surgeon doesn't call, so you have no clue if the op was a success or a resounding plonk like the others. Having done your Uber-taxi bit at stupid o'clock in the dawn time, you are very tired and lying on your bed at this point, trying to stay awake in case the pick-up is on again. You are well in the knowledge that the insurance has not approved this hospital stay and may kick him to the kerb at will, perhaps at midnight after the concert is over, as it were.

The final word is that he has lost too much blood – surgeon still awol – and that he has to stay in overnight. (Am I a bad wife for worrying that the insurance won't cover this illicit stay?) You are exhausted. You still don't know if he is any better, or what will be required next. The service of the medical industry has entirely gone out of the window – there is no handholding, no bedside manner. Just silence.

I get the patient home and he is very sore and very tired. He sleeps and sleeps. You imagine that this is nature's way of fixing him and you encourage it. You try to be a good nursey-wife, even if, in the back of your mind, you don't remember signing up for this and you know you are not very good or remotely qualified. You try not to wretch at the blood-colored bandages around the place and act willing when the dressing needs to be changed and the antiseptic cream applied. He asks you when your actual nursey-daughter is coming home and you wonder that too, since she actually did sign up for this type of work.

It's a big old dark place you are living in post-surgery; hoping upon hope that he finally feels better and can get back on the big old horse of work here pretty quick. Also, more importantly, that he is fixed. You also hope, for your sake, that your nursing *skills* will not be further required for the indefinite future. Wednesday, we go and see the man of the moment, the surgeon who did all this clever work to find out if it worked. Please spare a moment of silence for us old, wedded folk and our hopes that a new man will soon emerge from the hands of his surgeon, cured and ready to play husband again. Sickness and hospitalization are never fun; but they are especially not fun during the season of Corona and all that resides within her fickle world.

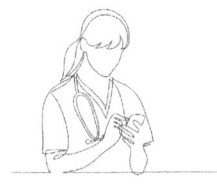

(2020)

Hope is not canceled.

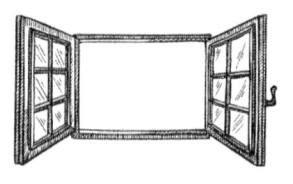

Friends of mine in England had so been looking forward to their promised Christmas at the tail-end of these long and tiresome months. After a long, brutal year of Covid-cancellations, they had been guaranteed a slice of merriment and celebration over Christmas. A little bit like a cease-fire during wartime; a short period when they could freely travel again and be with their people. 4 blissful days of delivering presents to loved ones and feeling a sense of freedom they hadn't experienced in a while. They were so excited and giddy with anticipation, that they could hardly stand themselves. And then, just like that, it was canceled. The feelings of disappointment were so much worse than they would have been had Operation-Christmas-Freedom been completely obliterated from everyone's minds when the virus had continued to surge; and people were still looking at each other and saying, 'They are still going to let us have Christmas?' Young and old continue to feel isolated in this new normal and, truthfully, a little desperate. There are health and work uncertainties. Money and security issues prevail. We are all spooked by this virus and the repercussions fly across the world from schools that need to open and teach our children, to the elderly that need contact with the outside world.

But do let's try and look on the bright side! (I hear my friend Carey's voice … 'Oh god, Lucy. Must you always be so damn cheery!') What is left? Oh, there is so much left. Hope is still there. Optimism that this will not go on forever and that, at least, there are vaccines being given out to vulnerable populations, as we speak. Okay this will not be a wonder fix for the world; but it's a start! As Granny used to say, we have to start somewhere.

Many have their Christmas trees up early and are enjoying the simple pleasures of twinkly lights and ornaments to contrast with dark days and darker nights. The nostalgic music from our childhoods fills the air within our houses and we are free to look back on Christmases past and remember good times when we were free to come and go, as we will be again. There was the Christmas I spent in the Black Forest area of Germany with snow everywhere, like a chocolate box scene; then the one in Paris so gorgeously lit up with sparkly wonder. The last few years before my sister Rosie passed, I would be almost skipping through Christmas so that I could be with her for New Year at her home in Turkey. She loved New Year with all its possibilities. Such lovely memories there. I literally just got prints made of those happy times from years ago and I will be making wall collages over the Christmas period. Already purchased the frames! Then there was the amazing

Christmas I had last year with my sister Mary and her family on the Isle of Man. I left California, picked up my dad in London and we traveled together to sister's island. Such lovely days were spent together. I still need to make a wall collage of those times. These are healthy occupations for winter lockdowns. I have already organized my book collection, so that they are not just dust gatherers and I can see what I have and what I am going to read next. Hope prevails that the next read will be even better than this one. If not, I will take the books to our local mini library and share with others. Now is the time for some of that too. Clean out your pantry and fill up the local food station. Do you really need 3 bags of rice and 5 spaghettis? I think not. Many others do. Is there someone in town collecting clothing as well as food and supplies? You can also cheerfully clean out your closet on a bleak mid-winter lockdown.

There have been too many broken dates in 2020, the year of complete and utter cancellation, that our expectations should be zero. Our family's presents are under the tree, and I tell myself that the worst-case scenario will be a revisit of Christmas around Valentines or Easter, when we will have mostly all received vaccinations and the world begins to emerge once more, bleary-eyed from the shadows of its covid memory. And that is the only way to look at it. It serves no one to bemoan our lot and wish things were otherwise during these crazy times. We have been taught some tough lessons: not to take freedom for granted, not to expect that Christmas can happen and family can gather. But we have also been taught that cheer is free, hope is free. You cannot always elect a certain situation in life, but you can choose how to respond to it. Let's start a movement to choose joy in this life of uncertainty! Let's put the sparkly lights on the tree and photograph the love in your dog's eyes. Let's take supplies to the food bank, knowing how deep the need is and how much people will quietly appreciate another's generosity. Let's choose joy over despair.

Christmas has not been canceled this year; she is just taking a quieter approach than the norm and teaching us what is important. If we are here, we are the lucky ones. We can speak, listen, breath, eat, dream. We are present. Let hope be our guide towards better days.

If you are despairing this holiday season, reach out to someone who can help talk you through it. Let them help you walk you through the darkened corridors, until you see some light that you can hold on to. "This too will pass," is what my mother said during tough times, and she was right. This too will pass.

Merry Christmas to all my readers and thanks for inviting me into your homes.

Peace, love and hope to all.

Lucy

Published in December 2020

International flying with covid

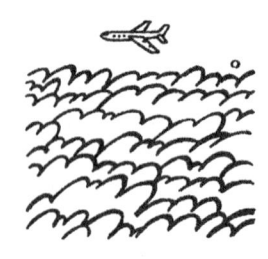

It was supposed to be just a distant memory by now; an inconvenient blink in the eye of all our busy lives and exciting plans. I think we imagined that, once the vaccine was available, people would be scurrying to get it, racing in their efforts to return to the human race. Some cannot for health reasons, and I get that. But many can and don't. The swift return to *normal* life has not been as most of us expected. Like an annoying relative, this pestilent plague refuses to die. It's still very much present in our every day, not to mention our future plans.

I have not seen my family in Europe since the Christmas of 2019, my father is 92 years old. How much do you think I want and need to get over to see my people? Much of last year was spent trying to book flights to get over there and being squashed at the gate. I lost more money than I can count trying to exercise my former freedoms to travel back and forth from America to England. This year I have been more cautious. Finally, once the passage to my homeland opened and fully-vaccinated Americans were accepted for passage without necessitating quarantine, I was all over it. I would finally be able to go and see my people. Hesitantly, I checked with my sister on the Isle of Man to see if there were any additional security layers I might not be aware of. Since that is where my dad and my sister both reside, that would be an important thing to know before I tried to get there. She thought the coast was clear, so to speak. I was in the driving seat again. Before the world changed its mind, I quickly booked a return ticket with my favorite airline – San Francisco to London Heathrow non-stop, here we go. Feels like normal life again. I almost danced. Somewhat like normal life. I still needed to purchase a rather expensive Covid 19 test – thingey – 4 boxes of tests in fact – test 1 -72 hours before flight, another test on day 2 after landing, test 3 on day 8 – am I dreaming, perhaps – but definitely another test before you leave the UK and one after you arrive back on US soil. That makes for a lot of testing – a lot of exams to pass. Also, there's something to do with a videographed test with Doctor Covid – who knows what that is – proving you don't cheat on your exams, I guess. No, don't open the box until you are ready to do your test. Luckily there is a helpline for the foolish like me, also probably most people who purchased the series of international box tests to try and get themselves overseas. Being fully vaccinated is not enough? Apparently not. I'm already a little afraid about all of that and how

I'm going to graduate my way out of the Covid box test without being arrested by the pandemic police and forced to do 5 years of hard labor. I digress.

I awake to an email telling me my outbound flight with my favorite all-time airline has been canceled. Outbound. Hmm. The return flight is still proceeding at this time. I gulp. My father is already getting the sheets changed for me at his home. Have to get there, have to. "Sorry, Ma'am. There are no other flights we can offer you." No other flights? Am I supposed to catch the boat home? I rush onto a popular flight app that I anticipated would show me oodles of choices for my chosen flying day. Not. Plus, the prices had gone up immeasurably. Well dang it. I thought lots of people like myself would be gunning it for London town in September. Worried about the Delta variant? Well, fish.

Oh look, there's a flight via Istanbul. That is a good back-up. No? As a hub for all kinds of interesting places the world over, an Istanbul flight would likely not get canceled the way my Frisco one did. Or would it? I was in a bit of a spot. I needed to get to the UK. Never mind if I had to take a 14-hour flight, change in Istanbul and get to London that way. Knowing me, I would sleep the whole way in any case. "Umm, you might want to check on the quarantine stuff if you stop over in a red country?" Oh, my sister is always the clever clogs. Hadn't thought about that. Especially since I had already booked the flight. Gaaa. I would hold the flight just in case. When I need to be, I'm a British and an American citizen. Which passport would you like?

I checked around again. Ah, Frisco to LA on my fave airline. Layover, change planes and then LA to London. Oh now, that is an undoubtedly improved option. It's a stupid o'clock flight, but needs must, as they say. I booked it.

Nearly a week before I am due to fly out and I am starting to feel pretty bold about my revised flight option working out. I call the travel company to confess I had made two bookings. That is what the neurotic do, when they seriously need to find a way to go and see their people. They book two flights. After an hour on hold with the worst music I have ever experienced blasting in my ear, the nice lady with a very thick accent informed me – I think – that in the case of duplicate bookings, that is a very bad and naughty thing to do, and you will be punished. Also, you don't get your money back. I explained my dilemma, but she didn't care. So now I only have one flight booked. Almost every hour of the day, I am checking to see if the outbound leg has been canceled. My inbound is holding fast. At this point. My covid testing boxes are smiling at me from their safe position on the bookcase and I still don't have an enormous amount of faith that I will get to see my family and my people in the coming days. I'll be sure and let you know what happens about that.

(2021)

No need to quarantine here

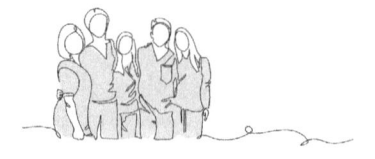

It seemed as if it should be simple enough. Used to be that way. I wanted to go to my hometown of my home country and sprinkle the ashes of my oldest friend's mother on the sea wall, where we used to hang out when our two families were together by the sea moons ago.

With all the covid restrictions still in place, (no benefit yet to being fully vaccinated) I researched how difficult that might be. The USA is still in amber status – though perhaps California should be already green – and that means certain rules and regulations must be followed for international travel. Firstly, there are airplanes in the sky – not many routes, but still, they are flying. The rules are that you must have a negative PCR test 72 hours prior to your flight. Can do. Then you must designate your chosen quarantine place for 10 days. No problem. (I need to finish writing my book anyway.) You would also need to pre-pay, book and show proof of negative covid tests on days 0-2, 8 and 10. If you would like to pay an extra fee on day 5 and that is a clear result, you will be free to go, but still required to get tested on day 10. My head was buzzing as I tried to absorb all this information. Oh, and the lines are several hours long to get through British customs. In this instance, there is no benefit to having my British passport and global travel status. Well, heck. I guess we won't be giving Jean a sea wall send-off anytime soon.

I haven't seen my people in over 18 months and that is a very long time for a gypsy like me. 30 years plus, I have been traversing the pond and it's currently very difficult for me to live as I please. I'm going to sit on that travel idea a while longer; at least until we are in green status and the passage home won't be, hopefully, quite so painful.

Endeavoring to look on the bright side, I remembered that we are not on lockdown anymore and I could go somewhere, do something different, even though it wouldn't be abroad. My daughter works part-time over on the Peninsula, and I thought it might be a bit marvelous for her not to have to leave the house so early on those particular days. We could just stay right there! You can forget how blissy that coast is when it's only a skip away. Ordinarily, I will only visit if we have people to stay; but that has been a super long time in covid land, and why not just go over there as a tourist? We all know how tough the hospitality industry has had it these past several months; do something helpful for those in your backyard! Eat some of that yummy fresh fish and chowder, enjoy those amazing views and listen to the legendary bark of the sea lions! Additionally, it's a great tonic to be able to relax in a motel room after a day's walking around and not to have to worry about driving home. I love to wake up to the sounds of sea birds and a salty waft.

We stayed a little off the beaten track near Cannery Row, (check out any number of travel sites; there are lots of deals to be had) but close to everything. I found a new favorite spot on the Coast Guard Pier, where you can be up close and personal with the seals, sea lions and their cubs. The occasional otter will drift by chewing on a shell filled with something delicious. Cormorants whoosh overhead with fish-stuffed beaks. I was completely entranced by these views of a magical marine mammal theater right on my doorstep.

I prefer not to be a tourist when everyone else is, so I met my girl over there on the day after Memorial Day and after she had finished work for the day. What a delight that was with light traffic, plenty of parking. fairly empty paths, lots of nice restaurant seating (in and out), and a fabulous opportunity to look at this lovely seaside town with a new sense of wonder. We had ourselves a staycation, as it were, dining at local eateries and spending a little money towards our remodel in the local shops. I was saddened, but not surprised, to see several commercial vacancies and I'm sure the fall-out from covid will continue to be fairly extensive in the coming months; but regardless, there was an air of optimism and friendliness out there that I had not witnessed for a while. It seemed as if folks were royally glad to be back at work again and getting shifts under their belts. The traveling public was out too. We noticed number plates from all over the country. We have all got tired of sitting around at home – this will be a summer of cautious, but persistent adventure; I just have a feeling. Everyone was masked up and sitting where they were told (lots of spaciously placed tables) and I was glad that outdoor *parklets* will still be allowed for restaurants going forward. I think this adds a nice touch of color to say the Fisherman's Wharf and who doesn't like people-watching? We enjoyed tasty local dishes at Abalonetti's, Schooners, the Chart House and La La Lounge and went home with a long list of other restaurants we wanted to try next time. It was a splendid, restful staycation and I even worked on my book while we were away!

Though the current world situation is a little disappointing in terms of actually being able to successfully fly somewhere that requires a passport, open your eyes to all the places you are able to travel to, closer to home, and make a plan there for the time being. There's no point in raging against the machine. In time we will be free to move around the universe again and that will be a wonderful thing. For right now, take a staycation, just like we did and plan to again. As Granny once said, "a change is as good as a rest," For us that was a true story.

(2021)

Opening up the world

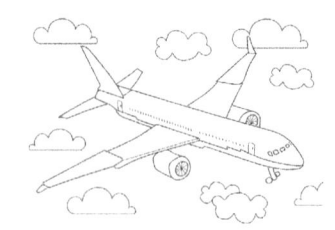

Two canceled flights and two covid tests later, and it looked like the US to UK flight might finally be happening. It would have to be via LA with a layover, but it beat the boat any day and I would take it. As the jet roared down the runway from LAX, I felt euphoric. I was going home.

I felt almost young again. Nicely rested in my lovely quiet hotel near Heathrow Airport and with another negative covid test under my belt, I was headed to the rental car place. I felt young-ish and free. There is nothing quite like the feeling of heading out on the open road in the heady knowledge that no one in the world really knew- or perhaps cared – where you were at the time. My day was deliciously uncharted with no deadlines. I had no responsibilities except to myself – a delicious sentiment.

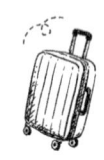

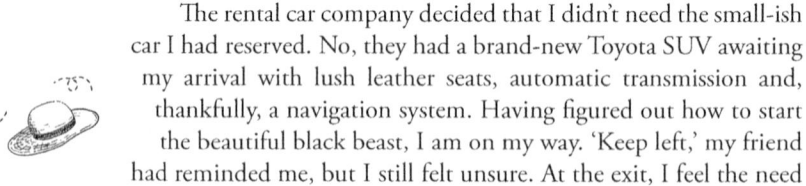

The rental car company decided that I didn't need the small-ish car I had reserved. No, they had a brand-new Toyota SUV awaiting my arrival with lush leather seats, automatic transmission and, thankfully, a navigation system. Having figured out how to start the beautiful black beast, I am on my way. 'Keep left,' my friend had reminded me, but I still felt unsure. At the exit, I feel the need to wait for a car to come along, so I could make sure I took off on the correct side of the road. All of a sudden, I didn't feel quite so young and free; I felt ill-equipped for my upcoming road adventure in England. It was nearly 2 years since I had been on that soil and likely 3-4 since I had driven over there. I turned off the radio and gripped the steering wheel in the 2-10 position like a rookie driver. I vowed to get there and all in one piece.

I won't say I arrived at my friend's house in the Cotwolds in a timely fashion, since I had diverted myself via my cousin's house in Surrey and paid her a visit, followed by a drive by to my aunt. These things always take longer than you think, especially once you get onto some good topics. It had been a super long time since I had seen them. The day was glorious, and I began to relax a little from my fist clenching. I eased onto the roundabouts like a pro and started enjoying the green countryside around me and the first hints of autumn. It was nice not to see corn-colored everythings for a change. The sun shone all the way to my targeted destination of Painswick, which is one stunning part of the world. My old friend and I enjoyed bliss-filled days of sitting outside in cafes and in her garden, visiting charity shops and catching up with our worlds. It had been too long since we were face to face. From there, I took the opportunity to cross the country – west to east – and scoop up a couple of days in my hometown, where, again, a heatwave welcomed me, and I swam in the North Sea two days in a row. My friend from the Cotswolds joined me and we couldn't believe our luck. England is so very beautiful when the sun shines! Since I had packed for more of a mixed-climate bag, it was fun to pick up a couple of more summery items in the sales and help the local economy a little. I was reluctant to leave, as I always am, but it was time for the last stop on my road trip – Oxford – back to the west of the country again and the home of another of my oldest friends. She and her husband treated me to a delicious dinner downtown near the colleges and I left the following morning to return the black beast back to the rental car company. She and I had become fast companions over the past few days, and I had even, finally, developed the courage to turn the radio on while driving.

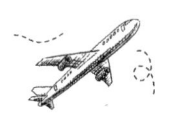

Everything moved along seamlessly. I had seen many of my people and successfully made my way to the open terminal at Gatwick Airport for the short flight to the Isle of Man. I had not seen my dad or sister in nearly 2 years, so they were well-overdue a visit. The Isle of Man had accepted my application to visit, and all seemed to have the green light. Traveling through borders in our newly re-opened world is not an easy thing to do – what with the copious testing requirements and the stacks of paperwork – but I did experience a blush of pride as I realized that I had just traveled – successfully – from the United States to the British Isles without skipping a beat. My sister picked me up and took me to her home where I was greeted with happy doggies and a fabulously comfortable hearth. We stopped via Dad's *palace* – also known as his bungalow – and it was so good to see where he was hanging his hat these days – so safe and well cared for. We spent several days cruising around that beautiful island and getting to know some of the lovely spots. The weather also gave us a wonderfully warm greeting which didn't hurt one bit. I flew back into Gatwick on a Friday evening and was greeted by another very old friend of mine who drove me to her home in the countryside for a splendid few days of catching up, eating delicious food and even river swimming. In three short weeks, I had crossed my home country a few times and caught up with my people. I was very content.

Now the borders of the world are slowly re-opening, the best advice I can give you explorers of the world is to read and re-read the rules and regulations of travel with covid that pertain to your destination. There were some very teary families in the departure lounge at Los Angeles who had chosen to not do that, and they are likely still tearing through their luggage trying to find those important documents.

I had formerly taken for granted my ability to freely travel back and forth from England to America. For 30-plus years, I had done so without blinking. Covid has taught me that freedom is not to be taken lightly and every trip taken is one to be cherished. Tomorrow is not promised for any of us.

(2021)

Our City by the Bay

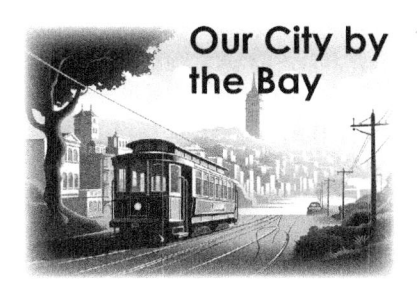

The last time she was here, there were young Asian girls wearing face masks in the elevator with us at the hotel. We thought they were a bit strange. Little did we know that the world was on the cusp of the largest pandemic of our lifetime. Days after that and we were all wearing masks and everything was strange, but not in that way.

Finally, she made it here. I warned her that things had changed a lot in the last two years, that she shouldn't be sad if a few things had altered, if stores had closed and the streets were just that bit more depressed. Our cities have not fared well the last several months.

I booked, what I thought was, a nice classic art deco hotel with a stunning 1930's entry way. How bad could it be? Hating to drive and scratch around for parking in the City, we left my Rosie truck at the airport and took a cab to the hotel. The first thing to be observed was not the beauty of the architecture, but the amount of street people crowding the entry way. A tiny Asian lady padded over to us as we rushed into the hotel and told us the owner was going to get the hose to rinse away the street people, as it were. Move them on to another site so the guests could enter the hotel in peace. Good grief, I thought.

"Where can we get some milk for our tea?" we asked, ever used to a nice set-up in our usual hotel room off Union Square. The café next door is closed, they advised. You'd have to go up to the corner market. Right-oh. Easy enough. We turned right out of the hotel and into a sort of barrio, where everyone spoke Spanish and several carried baseball bats. It was the opening scene from West Side Story – of sorts. Adapting our tough London postures of yesteryear, we armed our way into the *corner shop*, grabbed the milk and tough-strolled it back to the relative sanctuary of our hotel room. Wow. The Tenderloin is not for the faint of heart.

We were not going to be walking anywhere in that neighborhood. Fortunately, lots of cabs are available to be hailed. "Are you busy?" I enquired. "Not at all," he said. "The tourists have not come back. I'm thinking of moving to Florida." That made me a bit sad. My favorite city on the bay was lacking in love. The street people way outweighed the tourists, the local people were leaving in disgust. Empty store fronts gaped pitifully along the shabby streets. "DSW is gone!" my friend wailed. "Oh no, not Lori's. Lori's is gone!" our fave diner, the mainstay of many a year of visits and meals had left the building. Not even Elvis nor the classic car remained. We were sad upon sad.

We were happy, however, to see the good Japanese with the grouchy waitress still in place on the hill above the former Lori's. We quietly ate there and then caught a cab back to the hotel where we swiftly bolted ourselves in for the night. The next morning, the café right next to the hotel was open. As I waited to be served, I started up a convo with the lady who sat there peacefully at the counter with her little service dog. We talked about this and that, including her dog and mine. I showed her photos. It was all very companionable. And then she thanked me for chatting to her and whipped out her blind cane and found her way out. What a brave young lady, I thought to myself. Blind and acting like she sees as well as any of us. I started chatting to the barista. "I'm embarrassed by my city," he tells me. "They have to do something about all the street people and try to bring the business and spirit back to the city. I was born and raised here, and this is the worst I've ever seen it!" He went on to tell me that busloads of homeless people arrive in the City because of the relatively decent weather and generous welfare. The care systems for them are overloaded. Also, a whole other subject; non-sanctuary States send them to California with that whole NIMBY attitude. And then I felt really saddened. Our city by the bay was doing even worse than we thought.

But then I thought again. The soul and the spirit of the city is still there. As the streetcar ting-tinged her way by and a gull flew overhead with salt on its wings, I remembered how sometimes there is an appropriate time for resurrection – rebirth and hope – and our City was likely at the cusp of exactly that. More people are traveling now, it is becoming easier to navigate the world again with masks and vaccinations. San Francisco has always been a destination and will be again. The powers that be will find a way to better balance the accommodations of the needy and the residents and visitors. They have to. Things have really got out of control in that regard. It's no good feeling sad. We have to be supportive. I had considered maybe canceling our next visit completely. But that is not the way to support an old friend in need. My friend and I will be going back to the city to help her in her recovery. We will stay at our usual hotel and try to eat at our usual restaurants. We will visit the shops and do our small part in assisting the resurrection of our city by the bay, one dollar and one heart at a time. Maybe you could do your part too. Check out the travel sites – there are many deals to be had to participate in a few days away in our City by the Bay. The spirit of our city is still there; she's just a little battered and bruised. She needs you to show up and be present in her rebuild. She needs to know you love and support her through these difficult days. Let's be a part of the change we wish to see and begin the movement towards a better tomorrow. She's waiting for us.

(2022)

Secret Sisters

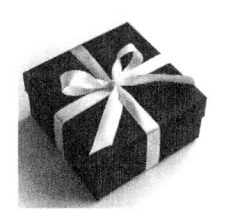

'Tis the season! Join my baking group, send Christmas cheer out to the world, be a part of a Secret Santa, Operation Christmas Child or Secret Sister group?' Normally, I wouldn't go there. I don't have time to be figuring out how to do my part, not let the group down, be timely in my attendance of the zoom meeting for the Pots and Pan presentation or any of that. But something moved me this year to do something that could be fun and raise spirits a little. 'Be a part of the Secret Sister Gift Exchange', a friend of mine posted. 'Let's start the Christmas spirit early!' Oh yes, that might be good for the sense of humor, I thought. It has been such a very down-spirited year.

I read my friend's message several times. I even made notes. Move number 2 to number 1. Don't forget to put your name and address on there, share ... Wait, did I do that right? Thinking I had finally understood the concept, I opened the door to my own Secret Sister Gift exchange online and the voices echoed back from across the world. People really wanted to get in the spirit early this year! A friend piped up from England, several from here, even one from Russia hailed back 'Count Me In!' My goodness me. I had a whole plethora of mature Secret Sisters all over the universe wanting to play a game with me. I better not mess it up! The weight of responsibility almost made me regret signing up, because it seemed a lot harder than it had first appeared. I messaged my original friend for guidance and created a new online group titled 'Christmas Cheer'. Seemed as if it would be better if we were all organized in one group setting. I felt better already. What could go wrong? Oh, lots can apparently in the cyber-group-sharing world, unless you are very militant and persistent with your flock. You also need to understand the rules. My group started to fall apart very quickly. Folks dropped out because they feared – with some probability – that no one would want to pay mailing costs to their country, others fell at the starting line because they found it more difficult that was originally perceived; and then they got so annoyed by it they ran screaming, as it were. The Festive Secret Sisters group was now becoming kind of a burden.

But then I saw all the festively decorated trees appearing online; illegal pre-thanksgiving decorating was going on across the country, post Halloween sparkle was popping up all over the planet. People, the world over, were looking for an early Christmas in their hearts. They wanted the sparkly lights, the music, chunks of goodwill to all men, the feelings that everything is going to be alright, if you have hope in your heart. Well, gosh darn it. If our Secret Sisters wanted a gift exchange, I would bring it to them and make it happen, regardless of my failures as a group leader. My childhood friend in Russia had backed out, because she felt no one would want to participate with her and her substantial mailing cost. Forget that. "Do you have Amazon?" I asked her. She told me she had never used the service, but it existed. I figured out how to order her a copy of my book, (via Amazon.UK is apparently the way to go), included a nice festive message and paid the $40 additional postage it took to get the gift to her. She was so delighted. I told her it was about time I sent her a present; we had only been friends for about 57 years! She told me she would be returning the favor. A gift from Russia – how exciting! We had such a lovely dialogue; I felt the holiday spirit soar in my heart. My friend in England said she could no longer play, because she just lost her job and must watch her pennies. Forget that! I shipped her a copy of my book too with a nice message. "I've sent you something just for wanting to be cheerful and play along!" "No way!" she responded. "That is so cool!" We were at school together over 40 years ago and haven't shared a gift between us since. This is so fun. I was on a roll and feeling light-of-heart and champagne-cheery. My dad told me his friend in London was on lockdown again and had just lost her dog. How sad! I sent her a book too with a nice message. She was so happy; she called my dad just to tell him.

You can find joy in some very unusual places. Sometimes it is under the tree, sometimes it's over the phone and, every now and then, it can be disguised as an annoying group game that blossoms into some severely needed world cheer. Never mind I got a random, possibly regifted pair of pink socks for my Secret Sister gift that made me laugh quite a lot. It is all about the giving – as Granny would say – and I don't mind a bit. I'm thinking that a proper tree will be in order this year with lots of decorations and lights. We shall put it up early and enjoy the bejeebers out of it through the holiday season and maybe beyond. I've decided to clear out the fireplace and put lovely sparkly lights in there, since we never light a fire, (I have year-round birds that sleep in my chimney.) How cheery will that be?

If you're feeling the winter doldrums nestling on your shoulders and you've got no appetite for playing a secret sister game, think about my story and how one small outreach can take you to marvelous places you never dreamed of.

(2020)

Soap and Water

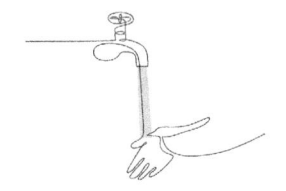

In January, my friend and I were up in San Francisco. We couldn't understand why so many Oriental people were wearing masks. Was this a new trend? Some were quite decorated and flashy. It was curious though. A little later, the reality hit. It was all about the so-called *corona virus*. The fear hadn't really arrived in our neck of the woods quite yet. When various strains of the flu are prevalent, you see the old masks come out and you see the warnings for the more vulnerable in society. That seems to be an annual thing; but this?

What on earth was going on? Had I forgotten it was some key holiday? Had we traveled forward in time, and it was the day before Thanksgiving? Could happen. Friday afternoon at the grocery store was never this manic. People were pushing around carts stacked with water and toilet paper, shelves were emptying quickly. There were long lines – not usual for that time of day. I was just there for my usual bread and milk, cheese and fruit for the weekend. I asked the checker. "Oh, it's the coronavirus," she says calmly and continues to check me out without further ado. "All the stores are dealing with it. I heard that Costco is a zoo!" Well, blow me down with a feather. A grocery store in Soledad is experiencing panic buying! Who knew. I went to the pharmacy where I experienced what I can only describe as price-gouging. $8.29 plus tax for a tub of wet wipes, really? They were running out of them too.

Back in Europe and the same thing is going on. My father is afraid to go to the shops. He's also afraid not to go to the shops in case they run out of everything, and he'll starve to death. He can no longer drive, so he worries about food delivery places not taking on any more customers. I read that Italy is attempting to close down and restrict movement to their population. These are unprecedented times, for sure; but how much of this frenzy is created by the media and the immediacy of all the information we are required to receive all the time? I hate to be casual about a pandemic, but the world is going nuts right now and that is not slowing anything down in the virus arena.

I contact my friend who was flying to Ireland, also Holland this past weekend. She sent over a photo of people basically wearing enormous clear plastic bags at San Francisco International. It was a bit laughable. When she arrived at her destination, she commented how everything seemed very calm and relaxed with not a mask or plastic bag in place. Perhaps that is just the Irish philosophy for you, topped up with the odd pint of Guiness! Maybe they are not as 24/7 news-frenzied as we are over here.

You don't really know what to think. "Wash your hands!" The serious television commentary goes on. Seriously? Who doesn't wash their hands several times a day? This should not be a new thing. "Use soap and water!" What? "If you think you are unwell, stay at home!" Excuse me? I assure you I am not making light of the situation, but some of the things I have read or hear are just – to coin an English phrase – *bonkers*! We learn this stuff in kindergarten or before, and I would hope that most of us are pretty well- practiced by now.

My father is moving to my sister's place on the Isle of Man this week – a small island in the middle of the Irish sea where there is currently no Coronavirus. He will be so relieved when he gets there. My friend and I have plane tickets to go to the South of France and Venice in the fall and we plan on making the trip. (How fabulous would an empty Venice be?) If the world is still dealing with the virus chaos at that time, we will be careful and we will be mindful, but we will still be traveling, if they allow us to. We will travel with all measures of anti-germ-catching devices, and we might even tote a couple of masks along with us. We will also be using the – not novel – concept of personal hygiene, washing our hands regularly with soap and water and trying to stay away from any coughing and spluttering members of the traveling population who happen to be too close to our air particles.

I remember London in the 1980's. We dealt with the threat of terrorism every day. The Irish Republican Army planted many a bomb in our downtown and our parks with a goal of maximum destruction of human life. Trains and buses were not spared. It was a threat we lived with, but it did not define our movements. The attitude was that you have to live your life and live it freely. We went everywhere we wanted to, regardless. That is not to say that we did not pay more attention to our surroundings or watch for strange things along the way. We did; that became our new normal. But we still went downtown, we still used the trains and buses and lived freely.

After 30 plus years of traveling back and forth across the pond, as they say, I'm not about to stop now. I shall continue to go wherever I wish, where possible, and exercise mature caution, as I ordinarily do. I shall also make sure that I continue to use lots of soap and water.

(Postscript to this story – we did not make it to France or Italy. All of our flights were cancelled. 2020-2021 became a traveling wash-out!)

(2020)

Summer Travel Woes

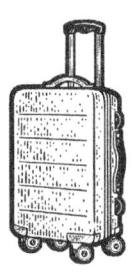

I am a British Citizen, born in Aldeburgh, Suffolk in 1963. I have lived in the USA since 1988 and have been a dual national and dual passport holder since 2003 without incident. I have always felt safer traveling the world with 2 passports and my passport renewals in previous years went off without incident through our British Consulate office in Washington D.C. Swift and efficient; that's what you want from a passport office. That's what you expect. You pay good money, and you expect good service in return. Until that doesn't happen.

And now this. I went online to HM Passport office, thinking that online would have to be an even swifter and more efficient way of doing business for my 10 yearly renewal. My first hurdle was the somewhat cumbersome *digital passport photo*. The first photo I took at a *Verified Passport Photo* department was no good. It had to be an *approved digital* photo and that is not a common practice for passport photos in California where I live. I finally found a photo lab that would perform one of those special things – naturally, for an extra fee.

I completed the form, uploaded the special photo, and delivered my valuable package with UK passport (that wasn't expiring until April) via the US Postal Service, Registered Mail.

There was a period of silence and then a text on February 11, 2022, advising that the UK Passport (Durham office) had received my application. Oh, I like this texting thing; I thought to myself. Very efficient! On February 12, 2022, the same text string reminded me to mail in my documents. Check. Had already done that. On February 26, 2022, I receive a message advising they had not yet received my documents, but to ignore the message if I had already sent them. Well, I had of course, but that is a silly time period when you have already mailed your important documents first class air and registered delivery. Finally, on March 7, 2022, they advised that the carrier pigeon had just delivered my documents and I breathed a sigh of relief. On Friday, March 11, 2022, and Thursday March 17, I received messages that they had emailed me about my application, and it was being processed. All well and good. I had hoped that I would have my freshly renewed UK passport in my traveling pocket and ready to go by March 18, when I was due to fly back across the pond again, but no worry. At least I had my US passport to fall back on.

On Thursday, April 21, I received a text that HM Passport Office had withdrawn my application. Wait, what? Where was my blooming passport? My application, my British passport that was still active, was now in withdrawn status? It was time to bring in the big guns and get on the phone – surely, I could get some answers there. And quickly.

Ha! I spent 5 hours of that very same day, being transferred from one department to the other at HM Passport office, because nobody could actually help me, or access my file in that department. No, they needed to transfer to me to someone who could; but I couldn't find that person. It was a nightmare scenario. The tedious background music gave me the heebeejeebies after a while; but I was very focused on establishing the whereabouts of my passport and, what on earth, after 58 years as a British Citizen without even a parking ticket to my name, could be the issue of my passport renewal? On the final transfer, a very nice Indian lady advised that the new law required that, if you hold a foreign passport in addition to a British passport, you must color copy each page of this passport and send this bundle of paper into the passport office to accompany your application. Could it be emailed? No, it could not. Could she make a note in the system, that I was unaware of this additional step and would be mailing said documents in to accompany my application immediately. No, she couldn't make a note. Would it be likely that they would be able to marry up these documents with my other now festering documents in HM Passport Office if I supplied my unique reference code? No, that was unlikely too. The most likely scenario, she noted very calmly, once they have withdrawn your application, is that they will mail your passport back to you – at some stage – and request that you start all over again. With a new passport fee.

It's now April 30, 2022, and I have received no further communication about my passport application. I was just reading in the London Times about the continued chaos inside the HM passport office and I am not remotely surprised. I am only grateful that I have a US passport to my name with a couple of years to go on it before it expires. Who knows, it could take that long to get my British one renewed; but I would really appreciate it if it didn't.

You must feel for the many people who do not have a 2nd passport to fall back on and who are having their holidays canceled because of this. It has been a long 2.5 years in most people's universe, and this is not acceptable. Horrendous stories are echoing all over the UK about families who are desperate to take a holiday and are not able to do so because their passport renewals are lingering in some moldy passport archive somewhere, surrounded by untrained workers who have no clue about how to help the ridiculously long lines of irate callers all seeking the same result.

If you are planning on traveling anytime soon and need to renew your passport, I would urge you to hurry it along with every dollar of expedited fees you can muster to accompany your application. I'm sure the US passport offices are struggling with these applications in similar fashion, though one might hope that they are not quite as inefficient as the systems I have been dealing with overseas.

    I'm about to start the new journey of PPRPart2 (PassPort Renewal Part 2) with a new fee – no idea why – in my quest to try and get my UK passport renewed. I have been a UK citizen for nearly 59 years now continuously. Truthfully, from birth. With all this ongoing chaos in mind, I'm worried that I will never again receive that passport in my hot little hand. Wish me luck.

Sincerely,

Lucy Mason Jensen
California, USA
UK and US Citizen. Dual National.

(2022)

The dolphins and the swans

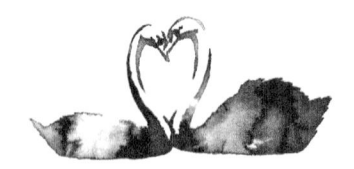

My goodness gracious me, it has been a very long 2 weeks in the history of our world! Since my last column, the world has gone from, *Be cautious, work from home where possible* to global chaos and pandemonium. Images, the world over, of overflowing morgues and empty airports have not helped brew any kind of optimism that we humans are in for a wild ride that has only the remotest chance of ending anytime soon.

Selfishly speaking, I had been looking forward to 2020 and all the lovely things I planned with family and friends. Now I am in no man's land, like so many others, finding it impossible to see beyond my own two feet, let alone my delicious holiday bookings in the coming months. If you had asked me what *social distancing* was a few weeks ago, I would have drawn a little bit of a blank and then chanced, *something British?*

The masses' panic buying recently in this lovely bounteous country of ours frankly made me puke. Those who saw fit to hoard toilet paper, paper towels, wet wipes and the like, should be forced to sit at home with just those items and nothing more. Lines of shoppers around the grocery store buildings with their carts also made me queasy. This is the land of plenty – there will be enough for all, but not if you act like that. I started feeling very ill towards my fellow man and dug around in my food cupboards in order to make do and not join that awful line. I bought bare essentials from the smaller markets that could use the help.

My father in London, not known for his calm demeanor, started, for want of a better phrase *flipping out*. Sister undertook *Operation Father* and got him out of London just before the heavens opened the gates of bat-shit madness with this virus, and over to her island where she lives in the middle of the Irish Sea. Her timing was impeccable – I cannot bear to think of how his panic levels would have risen with the way Europe quickly became the center of the pandemic. Though there are cases on the island, they are isolated ones, and no one is currently being allowed on or off the island. He is being well taken care of, well-fed and watered. I am so grateful for that. Sister reminds me I will owe her – when I am able – likely for the remainder of my days.

In all the 30 plus years I have lived over here, no one has ever told me I can't fly home. Having 2 passports, I effectively have 2 homes; but it has never been advised that I should not fly from one place to the other at will. At one point, in all the difficult and near overnight planning of *Operation Father,* sister got a little stressed and told me she needed my help over there. I checked that there were flights to be had – there were, though flying was naturally not recommended – but that quarantine would be required for 2 weeks when I arrived over there – before I could see father – and 2 weeks over here again when I got back; also, the island where dad was headed was, effectively, in lockdown. No, I couldn't really get home. It was a strange feeling; a little like the one after 9-11, though that only lasted a few days before flights resumed again in the new world we found ourselves. These are strange days indeed. Just as those days were, but with a different enemy.

My friend sent me a message that dolphins and swans had been sighted in the waterways of Venice, normally congested with gondolas and tourists crammed into every inch of that marvelous place. I had planned – booked even – to revisit her this fall with my friend. Dolphins and swans. That made me smile, it also made me a little wistful. Perhaps our planet needed a reset – maybe we had all got so greedy and wretched in our fast, instant lives that we would soon blow up into smithereens if we were not forced to slow down, stop, breathe, think, look, consider, stop.

Our governor mandated a *Stay At Home* order in California … no unnecessary travel or visiting, no groups of any kind. Restaurants, bars, theaters, and events are all closed and canceled. The world was closing and canceling; it felt a little like the closing of the planet, but then it didn't. I started to see random acts of kindness. People offering to go shopping for others, those with more delicate immune systems, the elderly, the young. Folks started looking out for each other again; there was a pause in the hoarding and gnarly behavior, a re-set in humanity, if you like. People began to thank those on the frontline of the tough work, those who couldn't shelter at home – and I must give thanks to all the healthcare workers and especially our daughter Francoise who is dealing with daily cases of more Covid-19 patients in her hospital. Thanks to the grocery workers, who have been trying to keep the shelves stocked and the tempers calm. Thanks to all the first responders who don't get to stay home ever. People started to thank other people again. This was a good thing.

Instead of feeling like the end of the world, it soon felt as if we were heralding a rebirth of sorts, spring in a very real sense; the spring of humanity. As the wildflowers bloomed and the river flowed through our valley, I felt renewed optimism that we would eventually get through the war with this unknown, but persistent viral enemy; that we would come through to the other side of our battle nicer, kinder, better; that we would be ultimately able to travel and live freely again. Just not today; and likely not tomorrow. All our precious plans would likely be put on hold while we followed orders, practiced social distancing, (easy for British people; don't touch me), acted carefully in our daily duties of life that might be considered necessary and enjoyed the benefits of our modern-day life that have not gone the way of my May flights or my April theater tickets. I can still FaceTime Dad and sister on their island. I can send a parcel for his birthday. I can still freely communicate with my beloved peeps all over the planet. I just cannot go there – at the moment. I will go there again, when I can. For the impatient and the free, this news directive is not an easy pill to swallow; but it's the state of our world right now and needs must, as Granny would say.

    Husband and I have started cleaning up our property. He planted a garden, (I supervised), and we started trashing out years of junk left abandoned all over the place from when we were too busy to pay attention and always planning to go and do more interesting things. This is our time for a re-set at our house. This is when our tedious work gets done and our small world becomes clean once more. We are all, separately, on a timeout from the universe and it's not all bad. The image of the dolphins and the swans continues to make my heart sing. The lives we enjoy will come back to us eventually. Just not today.

(2020)

The Lucky

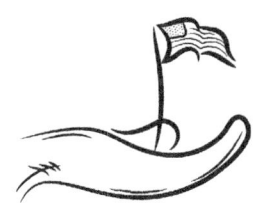

It has been a most interesting year; what an understatement. I have never felt so fortunate and yet frustrated. I have found skills I didn't think I had. I have dug deep for patience I never believed I possessed. 4 years ago, I decided to become a Notary Public to cover some of the gaps in my main job, real estate, that can be fickle at the best of times. I did the Notary and loan signing course and got ready to receive lots of work and get well-paid. Anyone who knows about notary work also likely knows that there is not much to be had and it is definitely not well-paid. I was a little disappointed that I had invested time, not to mention money, in my new endeavor. That was until the beginning of 2020 – a year that will live on in infamy for most of our lives.

Since the title companies were closed and the world of refinance and lending was still moving along swiftly because of the superb interest rates, notaries were considered *essential workers* and in great demand. All of a sudden, I have a chance to hone my skills, sharpen my tools – and make some money. I found myself traveling all over the place from Paicines to Seaside in my efforts to keep money coming into the house. It was such interesting work too. From your basic refinance to your powers of attorney and out of state purchase, I really enjoyed all the new things I was learning. I felt fortunate – I was lucky to be an essential worker, to be able to go to work – and there was lots of it to be had. How fortunate was I! Others, the world over, are well less privileged. They are forced to rely on the kindness of the federal government to keep the money coming in and the wolves from their door. I realized that, when life gives you a hand up, you'd better seize on it with both hands and be grateful – even if you are extremely tired. My son in Sacramento has been waiting for his fine dining restaurant to re-open. Not going to happen anytime soon. He would much rather go to work than receive a handout, contrary to what is often flouted by politicians. He has received a forbearance on his mortgage for a period of time, but he will never be able to catch up and pay the amount owed, unless he is able to work. He is stressed and terrified that he will lose his house. He is not one of the lucky ones. I hope to be able to help him; but husband has not been able to work either, so we are struggling too. There are many, many families out there like ours.

I travel to Salinas to collect Fedex supplies for my work. They seldom leave us supplies in our drop box locations. There are lots of people in line, no supplies in sight. I wait patiently for my turn and am greeted by a very huffy guy who didn't want to give me any supplies. He told me I needed to apply for them online. I told him, very politely that I was just trying to do my job and he snapped at me "how do you think I feel?" As one of the essential workers, I would think that a Fedex worker would be bending over backwards to be polite and helpful to their customers. After all they are still receiving their full pay and benefits and likely overtime with all the demand. I was so disappointed in that exchange, I decided to write about it. If you are an essential worker and you are tired, be grateful for your blessed opportunity to be out there and working and not stressing about your bills and your mortgage! I tell everyone who will listen how fortunate I feel to be able to do extra notary work when real estate is so unpredictable, and we are in the middle of a pandemic. The lady at the Prime shop in Greenfield could use some gratefulness too. She never looks at you or smiles when you go in. You feel like an inconvenience to her day. She is one of the essential workers too and should make me want to go into what I call my *fruit shop* instead of not.

The flip side of the coin was our visit to a business that is making the best of a tricky situation. I was driving to a notary job in Greenfield, and I noticed a very attractive situation where a restaurant had set up their outdoor dining space in former parking areas adjacent to the business. The flowers and fairy lights made for a very welcoming environment. *El Rinconcito* on El Camino Real had indeed taken the lemons from life and made lemonade. I could see that even from a distance and I pledged to take my husband there on a lunch date. We were not disappointed. The wait staff was friendly and welcoming, the outdoor dining set nicely back from the road and the wind and the menu delightful. My shrimp burrito ranked up there with the best of them and we pledged to return. "Yay, we've found our spot!" my husband noted, imagining how nice it would be in the early evening with the pleasant lighting and ambiance. I'm sure they will do extremely well, and they deserve to. They have accepted the rules of the new normal and turned it into an opportunity. That is what we have to do. We are lucky if we have the opportunity presented to us to take another path, explore a different avenue, make the best out of a tricky situation. For the guy in the Fedex, shame on you. Be grateful, be happy, covet the business income and security you are currently enjoying. To all those folk stressing on how they are going to make their mortgage or pay their child support, hold tight to the thought that there are many others out there like yourself and, surely, the powers that be will not want the entire economy to crumble to its knees. They will have to defer your mortgage payments to the end of the life of the mortgage, or something sensible like that.

For my part, I shall always consider myself lucky that I was able to keep working through the pandemic and maintain some semblance of normality during those tricky times. If you are also an essential worker, consider your lot and be happy. Try to be cheerful to others and make them feel welcome and important when they enter your business.

(2020)

The Masked Truth

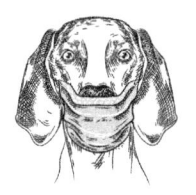

I had been looking forward to 2020. At Solace, we were going to be empty nesters for the first time ever, work seemed positive, we had lovely trips planned – places to go and people to see, both here and abroad. I'm not ordinarily a fan of New Year with all her fireworks and chaos, but this year – I have to say – I did feel a glimmer of hope in the *Auld Lang Syne* and the prospect of a better year than I've had in a while.

My friend and I were in San Francisco in early January, as we are wont to do. It is by far the best time to visit that popular spot and the winter sales in the shops are pretty good too for avid shoppers such as us. We stayed in a nice hotel off Union Square and remarked to each other how, everywhere we went, so many Asian people were wearing masks. 'Must be in preparation for a bad flu season!' we noted. Little did we know what was going on in that part of the world and how quickly it was headed for ours.

Early March and everything was going South in the world, such as our generation had never experienced before. Businesses were closing, people stopped traveling and moving around – there was an air of near panic on the planet. The virus was raging out of control in some areas of the globe and starting to make a huge impact in others. My friend and I went to have a massage and lunch to celebrate her birthday and we understood that the massage therapy salon would be closing after that day indefinitely. There was an under-riding feeling of unease – near fear – of what was really going on and what could possibly happen next. We had a good day, but distinctly felt as if that might be our last day of free living for a while. That turned out to be true.

April is a blur of shutdowns, lockdowns and whatever other kind of down we might describe. My family was also down in a different way since my husband was not well and his condition did not look like an easy fix. Fortunately, my sister was able to rescue my father from London right before borders closed and she took him over to her island in the middle of the Irish sea, which, in retrospect, was the best thing ever. He would have been so vulnerable and afraid on his own in London. And that would have created the most unthinkable nightmare – her stranded on an island and me on lockdown over here, with father doing his best to manage on his own. I was so grateful for her intervention. My planned customary trip to England in May to celebrate my Dad's 91st birthday was canceled – not by me, but the airline. In all the years I have lived in the US, this had never happened to me. Even after 9/11, the airlines were only grounded for a short while and then routes resumed. This did not happen in 2020. People were staying at home, leaving only for necessities; whole fleets of planes were grounded. The looting of the grocery stores for basic essentials was absolutely insane. At the beginning of the stay-at-home order, I was naïve and couldn't understand why the shelves in our local store were so empty. I'd never seen that before in America, the land of uber-plenty.

"Oh, it's the Corona," the cashier commented casually. Toilet paper, paper towel, wet wipes and hand sanitizer became coveted items that you simply could not find. It really was the most bizarre time. We went from the luxury of a free society with ample everythings to a state of lock down where toilet paper was a precious commodity and wet wipes rationed.

Then it became clear that this virus was affecting every part of life in every part of the globe, and this was a situation to take very seriously. It was not going to just go away; we would likely be dealing with the pandemic and its repercussions for some time to come and definitely until a proven vaccine was in place. We, as a people, had to become more cautious and pro-active to protect ourselves, our families and the rapid spread throughout the planet. We needed to stay at home as much as possible and away from other people. If we went out, we were to put masks on and exercise extreme caution in our sanitary habits. Wash hands, wash hands, wash hands. This seemed like a very smart thing to do, and I was happy to see the signs on businesses advising that masks were mandatory for entry. (It did seem a little strange, going into a bank with a mask on, but these were the new laws.)

I did not feel as if my personal freedoms were being violated, I did not question the science or the common sense of any of it. I purchased masks of different styles and colors to be able to coordinate with outfits and situations. I especially like the gaiter style you can just pull up from your neck over your nose and mouth. And then, in all the chaos of this world pandemic, I see that masks are becoming a political issue. What the? Some people feel that they should not be told what they can and cannot do in a free society; I get that to a point. But we have never experienced such a violent and aggressively contagious virus in our world – the numbers and the science speak for themselves. I fail to understand anything sensible that would make mask-wearing a political hot potato. I shall wear one for as long as it is mandated in our communities and likely beyond, when I am able to travel again away from my home. It is just the smart thing to do – for my own well-being, as well as others'. I try my best to stay well and healthy and virus free, but just like other inflictions, there is no telling who is going to be its next victim and I know better than to think I might be somehow excused.

Please, people. Just wear a mask. Make it part of your daily routine, like brushing your teeth or putting on clothes. If we can flatten the curve, we can then re-discover all the freedoms that we have had to set aside these past few difficult months. We will so much appreciate all of those liberties once we have them again; but for now, it's lock yourselves down as much as you can and be sensible. The science and the numbers don't lie! Please, mask up.

(2020)

The new normal

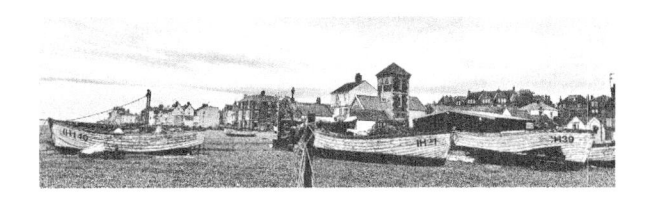

They say that when you do – or don't do – something consistently for 3 weeks, it becomes your new habit. I've tried to practice that theory various times in my life, such as a new exercise or diet regime. There is something to it. It has taken me quite a bit longer to change the manners of a lifetime. In a *normal* world, you meet someone new; you shake their hand and give them your name, by way of introducing yourself to them and vice versa. If you know someone well, upon seeing them again, you hug them. Those are the manners I learned when I was young (truthfully, the hugging came later; that was more of an American habit adoption).

Since the introduction of Covid into our modern world, people no longer shake hands and they certainly don't hug, unless you live in each other's bubble, in which case the odds are, you are so completely sick of being around them, you don't feel like hugging them. In the business world, I have become accustomed to either a brief nod upon greeting, or no mannerism at all; whereas before, a handshake was a customary and telling symbol of what that person was like. A strong, warm hand was indicative of that person's character. Cold and weak likewise. Overwhelming, ditto. It would now be very strange if we went back to how it was pre-2020.

I took my friend to lunch for her birthday – the first time in several months we had eaten together. I naturally went to give her a hug – she's my friend, we were both masked – she shied away from me and offered an elbow nudge in form of a greeting salutation and later a kick goodbye. That was weird.

At another friend's drive through baby shower, I had no idea what to expect. 2-4pm, the invitation read. Normally you would play baby games and then eat a lot. No one is invited into the house these days. The shower was held in front of the house with a table for the gifts, a chair for the mother to be and nice little plants as shower gifts for the guests. Not a chair in sight, no food or drink offered. I wasn't quite sure what to do with myself. I greeted the folks I knew, chatted with the baby mama and dad, and hurriedly left. That is no criticism of the event at all; I just didn't know what to expect and I felt unusually awkward. As we work through our *new normal*, I imagine we will eventually get invited into people's homes or offered a bottled water at least when we show up, vaccinated, to their parade; but I think humans are quietly embracing this new state of affairs, where gatherings are small – if allowed at all – (30 people max allowed at my friend's funeral, which left no seats for any friends only family!) No more the outlandish gatherings of all your best friends, lest you forget and offend someone, at least for the coming months.

I could have done with some of those rules at my wedding a hundred years ago when people just kept inviting themselves, the price per plate kept rising and my husband and I had to sell the classic car to afford it all. 30 of our most fave people would have been a much more manageable affair.

I have not dealt with even the smiggen of a head cold during the past several months. Not shaking hands with people, hugging or sharing air space, I believe, has strongly contributed to that. In the past I used to have at least one honker a season to put me in bed for a couple of days. I am now a bit of a fanatic about carrying hand sanitizer with me. If I can't soap and rinse my hands, I want to have at least a layer of security against germs until I can get to hot water. I don't think that will change. At one point at the very beginning of the pandemic, hand sanitizer was up there with toilet paper and paper towel in the rarest of items. Now the sanitizing manufacturing base has hit their stride and begun to enjoy their new popularity, there is no reason for any of us not to be armed with that magic stuff at all times. Check any lady's bag these days and you can guarantee to uncover at least a pack of wipes or a bottle of sanitizer.

It's become a funny old world, hasn't it! Staying at a hotel recently, I noticed that service had gone sideways with the arrival of Corona. You valet your own car and bags; collect any fresh towels you might need. No one will come into your room while you are there. The restaurant is self-service or take out only. You do wonder if that will ever go back to how it was. I honestly don't need my bed to be made or my towels to be changed after a night or so. I can quite easily use the valet cart myself and yet I do feel sorry for all those hotel workers who might stand in line for the few service jobs that will be available once the population starts moving again and staying in hotels. The cost of the employee might just be another victim of Corona that the hotels decide they don't need anymore.

One thing I am very anxious about is that our children get back to the classroom. That has to go back to how it was. My 6-year-old granddaughter has never known anything except distance learning, but she is not doing as well as she would in the classroom. She needs to start learning the social skills of a school setting, she needs to be able to play group sports and be disciplined by her teachers. When my husband and I were informed that our vaccinations would be set back because of the need to get all the educators vaccinated in our area; I happily stepped back for that. Friends of mine have communicated how their kids are suffering with depression and mood swings and that lockdown is weighing very heavily on their social skills.

Let's hope as the dust settles and we all become vaccinated, the new normal will see the children back in the classrooms and on the sports fields. I hope that there is a resurgence in customer service jobs and an anxiety to get out of the house. Other Corona gifts like hand shaking and hugs may, perhaps, take a bit longer to recover, if they ever do. I think I'm okay with that, as many of my British friends and family would concur.

(2021)

The nomad

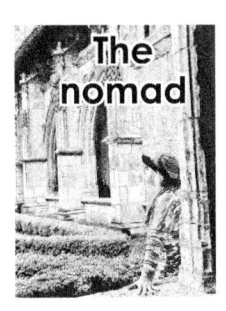

I'm a brat. There, I said it. I think my mother was the last person who said it to me many years ago and she wasn't wrong. I have lived and traveled freely all my life. I have cruised back and forth at will across this country and the Atlantic for 32 years now. I have 2 passports and 2 nationalities. I should be free to come and go as I please, in my opinion. And that used to be the case, before the *stupid-coronavirus*, (one word …. from the innocent mouth of my 5-year old granddaughter).

When my Mum was dying, I went back and forth across the pond about 5 or 6 times in a year; so many times, in fact, that my body no longer even bothered to feel any jet lag. It was just like 'oh this again? No problem …' Same with my baby sister. I traveled back and forth on that wretched journey (about the worst I have yet to experience), from San Fran to Istanbul and then south to Antalya and then south still to her home. The year she died I think I had done the trip 4-5 painful times. "I'm off," I would say to my husband, leaving behind – in writing – some very vital and, I'm sure, annoying instructions on how to properly take care of my fur babies, as if he didn't already know how, along with a couple gallons of milk and maybe a bar or two of his beloved chocolate.

It's a habit, a lifestyle even, that I enjoy. I have many special friends, not to mention family members who still live overseas, and I need to get over there and see them regularly. Not to say I don't love my family and friends here, but I had come to enjoy and expect the diversity of my life as a dual national and I had no plans to change a thing. Except Corona came along and reminded me that freedom should never be taken for granted.

May was my father's 91st birthday. I have traveled to see him every year for his birthday for many years. My old friends had booked a seaside house in our favorite place where I grew up. I had air tickets, even seat reservations on said aircraft. I was ready. *Your flight has been canceled*. There came the email; right after all hell broke loose with the virus in March. 'Contact your airline for blah-de-blah.' I was mortified. No, my flight cannot get canceled – I have plans. Places to go, people to see! But it was. It was not happening. August came along and we thought we'd give it another go. Try and get over to the old country and see the people, help my sister with the clearing out of Dad's house – 40 plus years of stuff in that old 3 story relic. She needed my help. Booked it and held my breath. 'Your flight has been canceled,' it tells me right before I was really starting to imagine that I would be flying this time. 'You won't be able to get over, sis,' my sister tells me. I hate it when she is right, which she is most of the time. Then, my girlfriend and I had plans to go and visit friends in the south of France. We had a whole itinerary. Fly to London, night in a hotel. Then fly to Toulouse in the South of France. Fly onto Venice after that … how exciting! My friend contacted me to say that, first, the Italian flight was canceled and next the French. Nooooo! Stop messing with me. It is very important that I get home to see my people! I have not been outside of this country in over 9 months now. I was very upset. 'We could get the train?' I broached. Yes, we decided. If my flight over to London did not get canceled, we would get the high-speed train through France and then rent a car. How fun would that be. We even had a backup plan to go to our place on the Coast in England, if it seemed as if France might be going back into lock-down. Yes, this would work out. Not. 'My flight has been canceled!' I practically yowled at her down the phone, like a cat stuck in a storm drain. I was so disappointed. America is a big country to feel as if you are trapped; but I did start to feel a little bit as if I would never get to leave.

Fortunately, my friend has just moved from Salinas and asked me to visit her in Vegas. Well, yes, I could do that without plane tickets that would get canceled. Easy-peasy. I would just drive across the state line. Then I pondered a little more. Maybe I could make a little solo road trip of it, stay by the coast for a few nights, celebrate the turning of another year and, maybe even, start proper work on my sister-cancer-grief book that I've been kicking rocks over. So here I began to plan my own personal bratty *staycation*. My own attempt to escape my life for a few days and be a bit of an independent traveler again.

My English friend, who is married to an American, tells me they are coming over to the US in November to vote. They will be staying in New York for a few days. "Oh, New York!" (My mind is already scattering around the place thinking how fun that would be!) And, here I go again, looking at the flights, pondering the possibilities. I am a brat; also, a bit of a nomad if the truth be told. I love to travel freely; I live to go places and see my people. I cannot wait until this *stupid-corona-virus* (one word) has left our world and we can resume somewhat of a regular existence. For my part, I already have plane tickets to England for late October and also Christmas. I daren't even think how upset I will be if the Christmas ones, especially, get canceled.

But we learn new things every day, don't we; even us old dogs. This *Stupid-CV* has taught me a lesson. Free travel is a privilege that not everyone enjoys. Right now, you do not have free passage to all the places you want to go; but you can go to Vegas, and, maybe, you can also go to New York. This year, I have been informed by the universe, more than once, that just because you want to do something does not necessarily mean you can. Bratty girl has been put back in her box.

(2020)

The not-fun-week

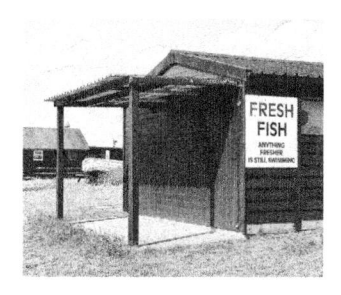

They said it was going to be really fun being home alone-ish (I have dogs). They said I would be able to write and relax, read and re-fill my spiritual cup. In addition to working and ranching and trying to figure out everything myself, it didn't happen. One look at Rosie (my brand-new red lawn mower who sat laughing at me all week) and the overflowing field of weeds and brush that I needed to attack in my backyard, and I was already in trouble. My Zen slid sideways from there on. How do you fill up Rosie, prime her or whatever? (He did tell me; I wasn't paying attention. Insert dumb blonde emoji!) Where are the light bulbs and the batteries? (Never mind – don't use that lamp much anyway!) Just as well the feed was purchased in advance, because I would have been in a world of hurt driving that beast-truck to the feed store, backing it in for the hay and all that palava. How do you cook the cabbage the way I like it? (I have been shown many times and still I cannot quite remember!) For my boiled eggs, how many minutes do I like them cooked and do you boil the water before you put the eggs in? (Insert another dumb and dumber grey-blonde emoji.) What a rollercoaster ride this week has been and that's before you even discuss hospitalization during the pandemic.

My husband was going in for open heart surgery, not a walk in the park. These days, you drop them at the main entrance to the hospital at stupid o'clock and then drive away. You are then at the mercy of surgeons having the time and inclination to let you know the patient has survived the surgery, whether it was a success or not and when he has woken up. 6 hours into the silence I was supposed to be enjoying, my imagination started to run wild. I saw images of him cut open and stone-cold dead on the slab. They didn't want to call me to tell me he was gone. They refused to inform me that the surgery was not a success and he had passed away. By the time I reached his nurse in the ICU, I was about ready to be admitted there myself; but she was super lovely and calmed me down quickly, once I realized he was still alive, and I was not a widow.

That was such a surreal time. And then he stayed in the intensive care unit, and I couldn't figure out why he still had to be on the oxygen. Why couldn't he breathe by himself? He went in breathing independently. What on earth had gone wrong? 'He has some lung damage,' they tell me. 'His valve replacement was a success, but now he needs a lung specialist.' A what? Mind goes gallivanting off again onto the south 40, as I imagine his brand-new heart valve behaving like a champ and his lungs collapsing. Gosh, the brain can canter off to some very random places when you can't actually see the person, touch their hand or look into the whites of their eyes. He wasn't even interested in talking to me, or texting. I felt so disconnected; as if he had gone away and some stranger had taken his place.

 I had a brain wave, as I was outside talking to Rosie, (still not actually doing her job as a mower.) He needed a soft toy and some goodies from the outside world to make him feel better. I didn't want to call some delivery service, I wanted to go and buy him a nice heavy bear to cover his eyes and ears, (hospitals are notoriously noisy places) and deliver the cheer in person. You are, again, allowed to go as far as the front door with your piece of cheer. They ask you what is in the bag and register it, ('No, ma'am, there are no weapons or drugs in the bag!) I drive the 40 minutes home quite pleased with myself and await a happy text. Nothing-nothing. Maybe someone had stolen it? It was a very lovely bear and a splendid piece of his coveted chocolate. Day 4 and he's still in ICU and still on oxygen. 'Did you get your delivery?' I broached tentatively via text. A few hours later, he replies. 'Yeah'. Well, that wasn't quite the euphoric reaction I had anticipated. What was going on? Who had replaced my sweet and funny husband with this monosyllabic stranger?

 They were all completely wrong; I wasn't enjoying this at all. I call to talk to his personal nurse, (that is a lovely feature of ICU!) I can't reach the nurse and husband is not replying. Oh, my goodness, he passed during the night. His lungs collapsed and no one wants to tell me, (this is a reoccurring theme.) I was frantic. Why would no one tell me what was going on? I call the main switchboard again and tell them my dilemma. (They must be fairly accustomed to near-hysterical wives on the line, thinking they might be widows.) They put me through to a nice, sane voice who informed me he had been transferred to the heart center and this was a good thing. I was so happy. He was still alive; I was not bereaved. However, once they are transferred, there is no private nurse – you are at the mercy of someone having time to inform you what is going on. Your beloved is on mega-drugs and has no interest in telling you how lousy he is feeling. I was really struggling to accomplish anything during this week that was supposed to be so fabulous, and Rosie was still sitting there laughing at me on the south 40, now neck high with weeds.

 Family members expected me to know what is going on. "What's the oxygen level? What does his surgeon say? When is he coming out?" Rapid-fire texts and messages zoom in from all corners of the earth and I am further agonized by my lack of knowledge. I talk to a nurse. 'They won't send him home on oxygen!' She informs me. Next message from himself. "I think I am coming home today." (Me: What?? On oxygen? I have my work all stacked-up today. Today is not a good day for any of that!) But instead, I sweetly reply *fabulous*. And then you wait and wait. And you wait some more. And you try to fit in the work you have scheduled with your north-bound journey to the front entrance. Then it gets super late, and the plan is that your daughter will go and get him. She arrives at the main entrance.

No, he is not being released, he just collapsed. Oh, my goodness me. She pleads with them to let her see him. Nope. She drives south and we still don't know what the heck is going on.

Finally, he gets home, still on the oxygen, but I've got that handled thanks to Lincare. Oh, and the commode they said I would need.

Meanwhile on the south 40, Rosie is still laughing. Thank goodness my son is coming home to take care of that sassy thing and her, by now, ridiculous weeds.

(2020)

You've been 20-20ed

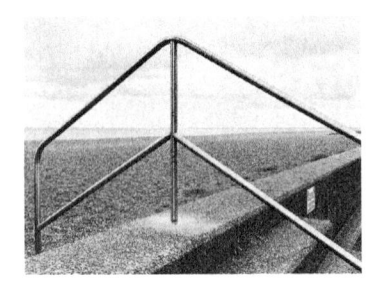

"You've been 20-20ed." It's a thing, likely to find its place in the modern vernacular, after a year such as this. Fresh on the heels of the ongoing Corona Virus plague, folks not being able to return to work, money tight and the future unclear; here we get doused in dry lightning and our fair State erupts in fire all over the place. We knew bad stuff would be headed our way when we endured that sleepless night, bashed about with cracks of lightning streaking across the night sky. Lightning in August is never a good thing here. Everything is so crusty and dry. We also had a fair amount of rain last winter, so the crusty dry stuff is plentiful and there you have an absolute recipe for disaster.

Fire, like surgery, is something that you become immersed in at the time and then the memory has a way of stifling the experience until the next time it pops up. I had forgotten what it is like to have everything covered in ash, day in and day out. I'd little active recollection of steamy burnt skies and the lack of proper daylight. The sinuses are bothered, and a thudding head is what you get for too much inhalation. You don't really want to go outside and, if you do, you are glad of your mask. Who would have thought there would be a day we would say that! Most of us cannot wait for the mask to not be a thing either. This is not the kind of Central Coast summer we boast about.

But one thing that has always resonated with me about the American spirit is how courageous and generous people can be during times of disaster. 9-11 springs to mind. Strangers helping strangers. Other terrible fires we have experienced here over the course of time – people step out of their daily lives to help each other, without money exchanging hands or an ulterior motive. It is so refreshing to witness.

This time around, social media has been alight with offers to help. "I have 3 trucks and trailers ready to go. I can help rescue your animals!" These people are not messing around and there are a lot of them. "Anyone need a place to stay, I have a spare room!" I have been reminded during these dark and difficult days why I really love living here. Taking the lead of generous souls, I offered our own fenced meadow on social media, aware that some people had nowhere to go with their larger critters. Within 2 mins or thereabouts, I received a message from someone I didn't know, asking for her friend. They had needed to move their horses that they boarded from the fire zone and the horses had been trailered all day long with nowhere to go. My sick husband jumps up out of his chair and whoops, 'yes, an animal rescue! Let's go!' They called me for our address and, within 15 minutes from start to finish, I had two beautiful paint horses rushing up and down my night-time hills, safe and free to roam. That is the power of social media at its best.

I love taking my lodgers fresh-fallen apples in the morning, listening to their happy nickers and feeling the velvet-silkiness of their muzzles. I have missed having horses in my meadow and it made my heart so very full, knowing that we made a small difference in their lives and the lives of their families.

Despite the continued awfulness of the pandemic that has touched every aspect of life, humans during our most recent crisis are maneuvering themselves out of the sanctuary of their own homes to go and help other humans in their times of need. People are delivering food and necessities to Red Cross evacuation stations and fire camps to cheer the tired fire fighters. Others are delivering pet food to shelters where people are forced to leave their beloved pets. We have all stood back in amazement in recent days observing the detailed logistics of a fire operation such as the ones that are currently challenging our State; and the confidence that the fire teams will, ultimately, get all the fires under control and allow people to return home – some to rebuild and others to clean; but home is more than just rooms and roofs; it is about community and humanity and communities are strengthened during times like this. I am gratified when I hear about the relative lack of injury and death despite the thousands of burning acres and I love it when I see the different agencies of law enforcement and fire working together on such a mammoth project. It really does restore my faith in the essential goodness of man, working together to help other men, women, children and animals survive in our fractured world.

We had forgotten about the last fires we endured and the fires before. We had all gratefully moved on with our lives, listened to the fire chiefs telling us to clear the brush around our homes and making an effort to do so, especially when summer comes along with her fickle ways and reminds us that there are many things beyond our control in life and fire can be one of them. Who would have thought that Mother Nature's lightning strikes would be the cause of most of these raging infernos all around us? It's 2020, after all, and we have been truly 20-20ed.

Let's hope that cooling ocean influences will prevail, that maybe we are blessed with some of the wet stuff to dampen the ardor of the flames and that something surprisingly nice happens in the near future for all of those in the lines of fire and the fire teams themselves. Witnessing some refreshing acts of bravery and generosity of man towards man makes me hopeful that something good will happen soon and many, many lives and structures will be ultimately saved.

(2020)

'And it never failed that during the dry years the people forgot about the rich years, and during the wet years they lost all memory of the dry years. It was always that way.'

John Steinbeck – East of Eden

SECTION 6

Just Me

Introduction to Just ME

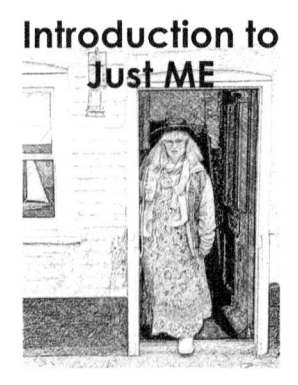

If there is one thing I have learned over the last several years is that you had better live well, while you can. People comment on my traveling habits. I'm always flitting back and forth across the pond to see my people; always planning for the next event. My attitude is that I need to do everything I can while I still want to. I see old dears being carted around on carts and in wheelchairs through the airport and I wonder to myself, will that be me? Will I still want to try and maneuver myself across the world when I can no longer do it under my own steam? I'm fortunate in that I still work, but I have a job share of sorts with my lovely partner, so we take turns to work and turns to take time off; and it's the best situation in the world. We share everything – even the good, bad and ugly. Especially that.

"What else do I want to do?" I find myself asking myself in the wee hours. (Lest I'm dying and I just don't know it yet.) "Where else in the world do I want to go?"

And it's not like I'm getting ready to pack up and leave anytime soon – I hope – but I think it best not to take the morrow for granted. That could just be me, of course, along with a few of life's invariable slaps and tumbles, that humble you in a second.

The section of the book called *Just Me* is … well mostly about me … and a few of my adventures from recent years, including a very large birthday and how I celebrated it.

Comments, advice, things you loved in this section? lucymasonjensen@gmail.com. You can't hurt my feelings. I'm far too old for that.

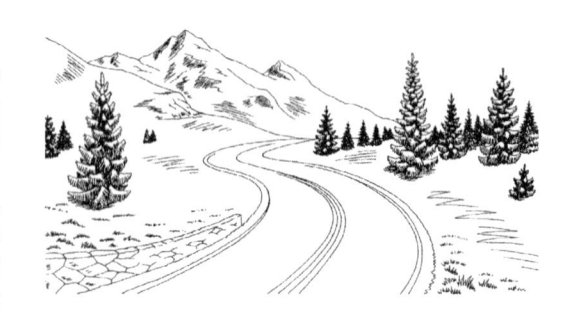

A New Adventure

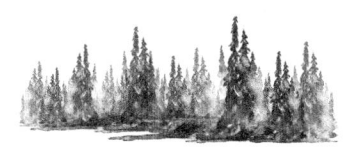

It all began in regular fashion. You are getting ready to go on a trip; so, therefore, things get really het up at work – not in a good way – and you are putting out fires, like California in summer – why does that always happen? Finally, you have put all to bed that you are able, and you are on the airbus to the international terminal, passport, and important documents in hand. Check. That is the beginning of a good trip. (There have been times when I have missed the bus; not such a good start!) You are cruising along listening to your music and enjoying the first vistas of the San Fran skyline, remarking in your cheery head that there is so little traffic on this sunny day. And that is when you receive a blocked call from the San Jose Police Department. Your world stops, though the bus keeps going. The driver had somehow left your case on the curbside at San Jose airport, and it could be now found nice and snug and safe at the Lost and Found, in San Jose Airport, while you were bombing your way up to San Francisco.

Funnily enough, I had remarked to the driver, when he was loading my bag, how curious it was that there were so many of the same bag in the hold – not just the same color, the same brand – you think he would have clocked that he needed to be just a little bit more careful. One would think. I got just a tad upset when I was informed about the fate of my bag, as we thundered northbound towards my airline with no bag in place. The driver told me he didn't feel safe with me sitting behind him, like I was going to clock him in the head or something as we whizzed along in the fast lane. At least he wasn't texting and driving at this point. The airbus company was not very helpful either. They told me that they couldn't really help me, except that they WOULD reimburse me for whichever service I found to collect my bag – or not. They couldn't have the next bus stop to pick up said lost bag, since they were not allowed to leave the bus unattended. I could not believe it. I was either going to fly without my luggage, or I was going to have to use modern technology at its best and have Uber pick up my bag.

The first couple of calls with Uber scared the drivers so much they disconnected the calls. Finally, Fahim in his Porsche Carrera took me on. "Oh yeah I do luggage pickups all the time!" He had a smiley voice. I could have kissed him.

I ate a little lunch with a large glass of white wine and waited for Fahim. Soonish, lo and behold, there was my black and yellow beauty sitting sweetly and fairly untarnished on the tarmac of the International Terminal. $107 later and we were reunited, just in time to check said bag and cruise through security. You would have thought that the airbus service would be checking in to make sure the bag and owner were safely reunited with one another? It was, after all, their driver's fault that he LEFT MY BAG ON THE SIDE OF THE ROAD! Nope. Customer service at its finest.

It was a lovely flight indeed after all that baloney. I had treated myself to a $124 upgrade and was very comfy, the plane being only about a quarter full. Arriving at Terminal 3 and cruising through passport control like a boss, or at least a British Citizen, I had some time to kill before my mandatory day 0-2 covid test at the airport. I enjoyed a nice flat white coffee (like a strong latte to you) and strolled with my lovely black and yellow bag in tow to Terminal 2. This is quite a long way since Heathrow Airport is a gi-normous complex. All well and good until I see the line – or queue – for the covid testing. Nooooo! I scream inside my own head. Fortunately, there was someone checking the thousands of people who were clutching their vital paperwork in hand and wildly hoping they were in the right place. I wondered, briefly, how many folks would skip out on that little mandatory requirement and take a chance that the covid police would not have the energy or resources to be checking that everyone had followed the rules. You can have thoughts like that after 10 hours on a plane, an 8-hour time difference and unusual bag dramas. "Oh no," the nice cockney lady tells me in her fluorescent jacket. "YOUR testing place is OUTSIDE the airport!" Outside, like around the corner? "Oh no, you will have to get a cab." Hmmm. The instructions very clearly stated Terminal 2 and not outside the airport. My wish to follow the covid rules was quickly waning.

I grabbed a London taxi and he proceeded to dump me in the middle of nowhere; a covid parking lot to be exact. I couldn't help but wonder how on earth I would find my way to London from here. Quickly tested (throat and nose, hate the throat part) and the parking lot director pointed me towards an alleyway, leading to a road, where I might be able to take a bus to take me back to the airport. At this point it was drizzling and my black and yellow bag was no longer feeling quite so light and fabulous.

I finally jumped on said bus where I proceeded to limp onto an underground tube station that would then take me downtown. Goodness me, what a palaver. Leicester Square was where my hotel was hiding, and I say hiding because I had to walk twice around the sizeable square, towing my now rather-heavy-feeling yellow and black bag, to find it. I asked the nice doorman at the Radisson, and he told me they had available rooms at his place, but I had already paid for my hidden room, tempting though that was, especially since it was raining proper by now. He did steer me in the right direction though – more than I can say for the local bus company – and soon I was in the dry. The first room the Victory Hotel tried to give me didn't have a window and I told them I couldn't sleep in a windowless room. It was upwards from there, however, and I soon got a back-alley room with an inoperable window. I had to be happy with that. I had arrived, I had my luggage with my clean clothes. I could take a shower and sleep a bit. What more can you ask for after that kind of adventure? Oh, you can ask for a lot apparently. I managed to squeeze in two West End plays in one day. Yes, it was that kind of a crazy vacation adventure.

(2021)

Carmel in January

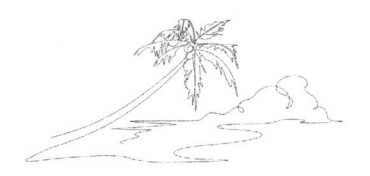

My friend from England comes to California every January. Most parts of the world are not that attractive in the deep midwinter, but Cali certainly has more charm than most. She can be wet and drizzle-mizzle in January – as she really should be – but my friend tends to bring the fair weather across the pond with her and I thank her for that. At least during the 10 days or so of her stay.

We started off, as we do, in San Francisco, the City on the Bay and, likely, my most favorite City. We have visited Frisco together for well over a decade now and we tend to have our little haunts we always frequent off and around Union Square, including a very good sushi place with a slightly grumpy hostess and, recently, Roxanne's, a cozy, friendly restaurant with terrific music near our divine breakfast diner Lori's. We don't even just eat while we are there. We shop! There are the annual faves – a 5-story Ross, no less, off Market Street. (Full disclosure; we have on occasion spent several hours in there and even, or so folk lore goes, purchased a suitcase to schlepp all our purchases back up the hill to our favorite hotel, The Chancellor, quaint and ever-reliable in style and comfort.) There's an enormous Zara, Anthropologie, Cheesecake Factory – more food – and this time, the delights of Tiffany's, which was not like Ross at all!

Her last couple of visits, we started and finished her stay in San Francisco, that delighted us all the way around. This visit, we have a tour bus booked with 'Painted Ladies' on an old VW Bus that we are very much looking forward to when we return there next week for instance; plus sightseeing adventures to the Beat and Street Car Museums. There's always lots to do and see there; boy, do we love it.

Next it was back home to the wilds of Soledad to pat the dogs and feed the washing machine – also check to make sure the husband is still alive. Not even making the time to unpack properly, we were off again, this time to Carmel-By-The-Sea, a divine spot right in our backyard. Years ago, when my mother was still alive, my parents would visit me from England and always stay at the Fireplace Inn in Carmel, no matter where I lived at the time. Gosh, they loved it. They had all their favorite haunts, places to go and eat. Since we live only an hour away, it never seems to make sense to spend the night, but having a friend to stay is a great excuse to do just that. We could enjoy Carmel for a day and night and swing by Monterey on the way home.

We arrived on a Sunday afternoon in radiant sunshine. Driving straight down Ocean to the white-whipped sands of that special beach, right off the cuff, we bumped into some old friends and their dog. That was very lovely; especially since I had fostered that very same dog a few years back. And then we came upon multitudes of other people and their dogs, all having the time of their lives. People were paddling, surfing and picnicking to their hearts' content. Some, like us, were just trit-trotting along the damp sands, admiring the significant waves of the King Tides and dog-watching like the dog-holics that we are. (Definitely could have stolen a couple of border collies from there and also a spectacular Ridgeback!) Where in the world can you do all of that on a Sunday afternoon in January? It was so delightful.

We had booked a room at the Carmel Inn, but our room wasn't yet ready, so went off on a wander to the village. We stopped in at the new Anthropologie shop in Carmel Plaza and enjoyed a cup of tea in the Carmel Roasting Company. Then it was time to consider where to have dinner later. Gosh golly, such a fine selection of places to choose from and all within walking distance from the Inn. You don't really want to keep navigating the parking spaces when you are visiting Carmel. Much more fun to watch your steps add up on the Fitbit and enjoy the delicious sea air. Soon it was time to meet friends for drinks and so off we went to La Playa hotel and bar, a beautiful twilight stroll with ocean peeks along the way. Their 5pm dime drinks went down a treat, especially since the Packers were beating the Sea Hawks, and we had a wonderful few drinks in that very special bar. From there, it was onto Terry's, the home of our lady Doris Day, for a few more drinks and appetizers. Such a fun evening to be had in pastures new, just a step away from our own front door.

If you are tired of the same old thing in January, the sadness that can permeate after the decorations come down and the still chilly winter nights, step out of your comfort zone and have a little *staycation* in your own backyard. Better still; invite an old friend over to share it with you. Walk along the beaches of your own beautiful State and feel the oxygen in your lungs. Be happy you are alive and healthy enough to get out and enjoy it.

Published in January

Going home again

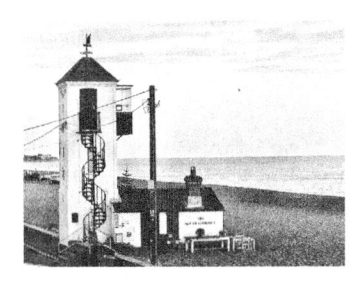

They say you can't go home again. Though it is certainly not for everyone, it's my experience that sometimes you can. I was recently fortunate enough to be able to spend a week not only in my hometown, but in my home cottage where I was born and grew up. Over the past 35 years I had dreamed about that place – mostly with my Mum, or in situations where we couldn't find the key (a recurring theme, since we never used to lock the door and therefore couldn't find the key when we were getting ready to leave!) I never dreamed about returning as an adult.

It was the most random thing that occurred. I was walking by the house, my old cottage, the last time I was there in town. Whenever I travel across the pond, I'm always drawn to spend time there, like a homing pigeon, flying on instinct. I always pass my old cottage and peep in the windows, for old times' sake. I knew she had recently re-sold, and I was curious if our old furniture was still there from the previous owners, who had ignored my requests for the old captain's chair my parents had left behind. This time, a lady was vacuuming. Ah. Ooh! Should I knock? Maybe she would let me see the place again? Maybe they might have plans to rent it out? Would that be weird? For some people, yes. For me, Queen of Nostalgia, it would, in some ways, put things to rights in my world. Losing my childhood home had never set right with me. I knocked on that old familiar door. A lady opened the door in a somewhat guarded way. That made me feel as if she was from the city and not accustomed to being disturbed in this fashion. She didn't invite me in, but she did tell me that the cottage could be rented out. I was a little bit exhilarated. I had never imagined this particular scenario. Maybe she thought I was a weirdo, as I endeavored to relate my story.

I talked it out with my people, my girlfriends, and we decided that it would be a super wonderful thing to rent this place. We had all spent chunks of time there in the past and this might be a rather special thing to do decades down the road, truthfully the year of our 60th birthdays. And so, 3.5 decades after I had been there for the last time, we rented the cottage.

Entering the familiar threshold was, truthfully, a bit overwhelming, euphoric even. I felt transported to another zone, a familiar yet unfamiliar arena of my former life. I had dreamed of being inside these walls again, but it had never quite felt like this. The cottage was, essentially, the same. She had the same doors, windows, thresholds, bones. Okay, she also boasted central heating, a new kitchen design and other bits and bobs, but basically the cottage of my childhood was the same. It took about the whole week to soak all of this in; but I realized, after about day 2, that actually it wasn't amazing anymore, or strange; it was just normal.

My mother's best friend crossed the threshold of the cottage to come and enjoy dinner with us in the backyard on a lovely sunny evening and she immediately teared up. Since my mother had died over 2 decades ago and it had likely been another decade or so on top of that since her oldest friend had seen her there, this was likely quite a momentous and emotional event. The decades fell into one another, compounded into a big old pile and, all of a sudden, it was just a few days ago that we were all there. Time meant nothing. "I wasn't expecting to feel this way!" Mum's old friend exclaimed. 'Actually, I wasn't expecting to feel any of this." And I don't think any of us did.

We entertained others in our cottage. Though the art on the walls was different, the furniture and the vibe, the aura within those walls was the same. "How does it feel?" my friend asked me. I could only respond that it felt 'thick', as if all the spirits within the walls were still there timelessly waiting, transcending time and waiting for me to come back – an experience you can only describe if you go there.

It felt right to have people visiting and feasting within those walls as we always had. My oldest friend and I sat at the old table – not our old table, but one similar – and we worked on the story of our childhood together, a project we have been working on remotely between Oxford in England and Soledad in America and now we were together again. It felt so right to do it there as if the creative juices flowed particularly well in that space. In our youth, our houses were right next door to one another, and we spent days and weeks in and out of each other's homes. Now our families are depleted and our home ownership no more, we still felt as if we were young again and on the verge of some marvelous lives ahead.

They say you can't go home again. I think I just did.

(2023)

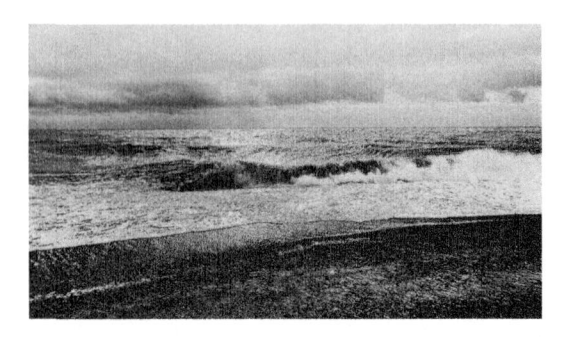

Gratitude

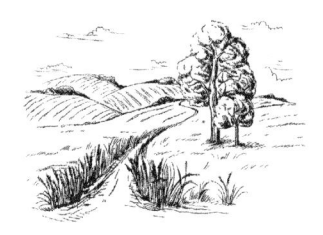

October is a funny old month. Some days are hot as summer, yet with stilled winds in the afternoons and an icy bite to the early mornings and evenings. November can be more of the same, yet the time of year is marked by the turn of the vines – the rich colors bending from yellows and greens to dark reds and near black hues as the darker days of winter approach. I love this time of year, though my body struggles with the changing temperatures and oftentimes fights a cold through the transition of the seasons.

As I drove across the valley, I was stunned by the array of autumnal colors – the swathes of yellow and green, then the fall vines telling us about the time of the year, fruit flies hanging onto the last drips of nectar. Halloween is just a memory of rotting pumpkins and seasonal décor leaning towards Thanksgiving, one of the most civilized dates on the American calendar.

As I crossed the green bridge onto Arroyo Seco Road and saw the whisper of the river still running, I felt overcome with gratitude for the place we call home, the beauty of the hills and fields, the blessing of the fresh airs all around. We really do live in one of the most beautiful places on earth.

And here we are a skip away from Thanksgiving. I recall my early experiences of Thanksgiving – the strange mixes of fruit and jelly on a plate with turkey and sweet potato. Pumpkin pie for dessert with a sweet-savory taste that I found rather bizarre. I may not have understood the combination of flavors, but I learned to accept them over time in my palate and enjoy the meaning of the season.

I do recall that people were kinder to us over Thanksgiving. Whatever we experienced other times of the year, there was a sense of calm gratitude that came over folk around the holiday that they passed along to others; a time to take stock and be thankful for all the plenty in their lives. I'll never forget someone trying to give us a Thanksgiving basket from the Salvation Army our very first Thanksgiving in Louisiana and I refused it thinking it was charity that we didn't need and not just the meaning of the season, sharing with those less fortunate that our neighbors thought appropriate for us.

I like hearing about food drives and free Thanksgiving meals in our local communities. It makes me feel a part of something much larger than myself. This year, the Soledad Merchants Association are having a Business Expo at the Community Center. The entrance fee is a canned good or non-perishable food item – or as many as you can afford to donate – to help the Salvation Army feed those who struggle to feed themselves; and as winter arrives in our area, there is a very real need for that. The crops move to Arizona and things dry up and hibernate here until the spring. I used to like to do shoe and jacket drives also this time of year to share with our local families. I often cast a look back to my first Thanksgiving over here when I didn't even have a bed or furniture to my name – just the shell of a rather large and leaky double wide trailer home on the bayou in Louisiana.

It's important not to forget those times when you were hungry, without, less than. There are many community organizations out there that can help and will equally receive help from you when you are in a position to give. Pass it along, I have said to people when they thank you. When you are able – pass it on. Don't forget the pets either! If families are having struggles feeding themselves, it is likely that their pets are more than left behind. I shall be adding some extra cans of pet food to the food drive pantry this Thursday.

When you look outside your window this fall, stop for a minute to examine all the beauty in our autumnal colors, spare a thought for those less fortunate and think about how you might be able to contribute. There are way too many families in our community who suffer food anxiety. If, like me, you currently don't, it's your responsibility to step up and assist. I could not imagine if my children were hungry. Could you?

I'll never forget the Salvation Army food basket that arrived like a surprise at my door in Back of Brusly, Louisiana on Thanksgiving Day. Had I been hungry at the time, that basket full of goodies would have shown up like manna from heaven.

We are so lucky to live where we do in the salad bowl of the world. When the lettuce crop and the summer fruits are no longer feeding the families that pick the crops, we must all gather together and add the help where the help is due.

It's called humanity.

(2023)

Home for the holidays

There is perhaps no better sound in the world than that of a familiar wave slapping against a familiar beach. I was born and grew up with that sound on the East Coast of England. When I return to my source it is almost a primal journey back to the essence of what I was and where I came from. I can sit and listen to it for hours, watching the eternity of the lapping wave – one after another they follow, the sea sometimes blending in with the sky, simultaneously changing colors like a moving landscape of steely greys and greens, blended with browns, that tells me I am home. It calms me and makes me whole.

I am home for the holidays, oft sang with sentimental lilt at this time of year; but it is a lovely time to be home. Though I don't own a cottage here anymore, I am so lucky to be able to rent my old home and touch the familiarity of its bones once more, feel the spirits of those who passed through and who were dear and still are. Wherever I go in the world, I am most grounded when I am here. I feel my soul be able to pause, slow, stop, sleep the slumber of an often anxious spirit. My daily world feels so very far away from here, when I am here; not that that world isn't wonderful in its own way, but here I can be a child again. I can walk along the beach, visit the landmarks, saunter down alleyways, pace the same seafront, sit on the same sea wall and I am me, but a lighter me, less burdens of work, home, responsibility, age – more me and that innocent little girl who grew up here.

My oldest friend and I just finished co-authoring our latest book – a collection of memories from our childhoods here on the East Coast of England in the 1960's and 1970's. We were charmed children, best friends, living next door to one another, able to run free on bicycles and on our little legs all over the place, with dogs and friends everywhere we went. In and out of the sea every day, out and in the friendly shops all over town, blessed with a rare freedom you just can't give children anymore.

It has taken us about 18 months of back and forth and sharing memories and pictures, putting them into some kind of coherent order and putting our manuscript together; she in Oxford, England, me in California, enhanced by her very considerable graphic designer skills. And here we are, very close to publishing our childhood memoir that we talked about and made happen. And here I am, staying just a skip away from the South Lookout, the sentinel of our childhood, the tower that was always right there next to where we were sitting on the beach, hanging out on the sea wall, swimming in the sea. It was always there watching over us. Now I can watch over it from my window on the world over the beach and bay of my hometown. I glance over as I write and sip and chat and there it is as it has always been.

Fortunately, the late 60's and early 70's heralded the early days of Kodacolour film that you could get developed in the local chemist and several people snapped our moments in time around the South Lookout that have lived on in dusty old albums in dark chest of drawers. Lizzie and I extracted these moments from her parents' albums and mine to bring together the color, light and life of those special times. We gathered together other voices who had come to visit during those years and gave them a place in our book as well. It has been a labor of love over several months. *The South Lookout – Our Aldeburgh Childhoods* is our story. Maybe it will inspire you to write up your own story – if not for you, then for your children and grandchildren that they may know you better and the era that you grew up in; not to mention their own heritage.

For some people coming home can be painful, reminders of things lost or left behind. For some the thought of staying in their childhood home might be more than they can bear, knowing that they never wanted it sold as it was. For me I have made my peace with all of that, and I am unburdened these days by wishes that things were otherwise. I am so very happy to be back home for the holidays in the knowledge that home is so much more than bricks and doors. It's the place where your people reside and gather, a spot on the universe where beloved spirits might collide and embrace you as you pass. For us, it's right there around the South Lookout in a small coastal town called Aldeburgh on the East Coast of England.

Our Lookout, Our South Lookout

Like an old grandpa, he was just part of the landscape
A place you passed, a spot you loved
You knew he would be there, always there, like scenery.
Unlike most things.

He was built around 1830 to help
Ships passing by.
He was the watchman
Of the bay,
The keeper of
Those in peril
On the sea.

As the stepping-stone to the beach and the water,
He watched all of us -
The sentinel of our youth.
Those times that you remember as
The very best of all times
In sun-kissed hazy memory
He was there.

*He saw our tea and ginger cake trays
After long days in the sea.
He saw our laughter and our stone seeking,
Day in and day out.
He saw the friends and the boyfriends coming and going.
He saw people dying and babies born.
He saw us sell our houses and move away,
Knowing we would be back
And we would be sad
It happened
As it did
For all of us.

He saw it all.
Our Sentinel, our South Lookout
Our quiet stone watch tower.

Even now,
He hears our voices, counts our steps.
He knows us when we come.
We skip over the sea wall by his side
And he welcomes us home.
However long away we have been.

We never thought of his aging,
The effects of time and storms upon his walls
We expected him to always be there,

Always present as our sentinel, our lookout
Like our grandpa and those before.

He kept our place on the beach for us,
Every weekend, every holiday.
He watched over the young
As they splashed in the surf.

He told us when it was
Not the time to test the water
Or its powers.
With shuttered lid in greys and dusk,
He kept watching
Over us*

The Look out,
Our South LookOut.
Our fine stone structure of great stature,
Historical and landmark
And personal,
Very personal.

Our old friend
Encapsulating memories of all those happy times
And the times before
And the times before us
And surely the times after.

Sending peace to you and yours. May you all find Christmas in your hearts.

Lu

(2023)

Late for it all

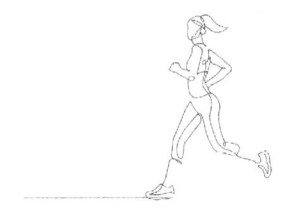

I don't know what happened. We skipped through Halloween, enjoyed a nice, peaceful Thanksgiving and then all heck broke loose. I took an early Christmas delivery to my dad and sister overseas – and how organized was I! Even had the holiday gift bags and tissue paper in my luggage all ready to be present and perfectly put together under my family's trees, (that were already up and pristine, glistening with the joy and hope for the season.) Normally I am scrambling to the post office to make the deadline for overseas shipments and then staggering under the pressure to mortgage my house to pay for priority shipping. But not this year. My large blue case was firmly packed and overloaded with all of their blessings. I was just that organized this year.

Then I got sick. Never mind I was fully masked the whole 10 plus hours of the flight. Something snuck in and gave me a nasty virus. By day 2 of my trip, I was hacking up a lung and investing in all measure of English cold and cough medicines I could to help me feel better. Nothing worked, except for, maybe the hot mulled wine for a little bit at least.

By the time I arrived at my sister's house on the Isle of Man, everyone was hating me – nearly as much as I was hating myself. Sister managed to get me some antibiotics, by way of the magic phone doc that talks to you and issues you a prescription, free of charge – but still the evil virus hung on in the lower regions of my poor old chest. Everything hurt! I went to bed and hardly visited with my old dad. It was a sad state of affairs for our early Christmas visit.

By the time I arrived back on US soil, still hacking and hating, I was so far behind with the holiday season that I might as well send out a *Happy January* greeting out to all and sundry, or perhaps an early missive for Christmas 2023. What happened to Miss Organized? She had sunk in the ship of good intent.

As I ventured to approach my office desk, piled with not-dealt-with crud, I noted all the cards I had planned to send, all the folks I had planned to thank and nothing was going anywhere on time. I felt like a complete loser. I know people who get organized in August, for crying out loud; what is wrong with me? Still the virus hung on like an unpopular relative, inviting themselves over for the entire holiday season. "You've got the RSV virus," my friend noted helpfully. And I realized that I likely did. No matter all the medicines I imbibed and the full course of antibiotics I ingested like a good girl, this beast was seeming like a keeper in my body. I was so over it.

"I'm so behind!" I bemoaned to anyone who would listen. "Hey," a friend sent over her cheer and understanding. "We are all behind. Everyone will understand. The most important thing is you traveled successfully across the world to deliver cheer to your family. Not many of us can say we accomplished that!" And with that, I stopped hacking and took stock of my good fortune. Yes, I did that this year. Never mind I forgot to send cards to you and you and you, you will just have to forgive me. I was sick with RSV, I traveled across the world – was sick – for many, many days – and I never caught up with myself. If you receive a New Year greeting from me, still bedecked with holly and snow and fireplaces of the festive season that was – I'm going to apologize in advance and pledge to try and do better next year. I've yet to unpack my bag from my travels, my laundry is in a huge pile smiling at me and my granddaughter will arrive soon, expecting her room to be cleared of my luggage. Plus, I still have the virus. Feel my pain?

Seasons greetings to all – this is the best I could do. Happy Christmas after Christmas, as it were. I send you a timely greeting of health and happiness for the coming year. At least I'm not late for that, (unless I miss my editorial deadline … could happen …)

Love to you all – from my home at Solace to yours, the world over.

Lucy

(2022)

Magic

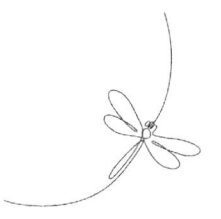

Very soon after Winston Churchill Sebastian Mason Jensen – aka Sir Winston White Horse – went to sleep on April 2, some funny things started to happen on our ranch. Previously, the llamas and goat were his hang-out buddies on the land below. They would move around together, as grazing animals are wont to do, presenting quite the most eccentric combination of hooves and coats. Neighbors passing by our 7-acre parcel would remark on my motley crew and ask how on ever I managed to put that gang together. Occasionally the 3 llama boys would come up to see what Win was chewing on at the house, since he loved to graze on the lawn and hang out with us and the dogs where possible; but generally speaking the boys were grazing well away from the house in their own rambling world, especially when the land was teeming with yummy things for them to gnaw on, as it was after last winter's rains.

As soon as Winston died, the llamas were not only up by the house, Harold Malcolm Democracy – chief llama – was positioned on the deck right next to the house. This had never happened before. The first several days after Win passed, Harold had the most eerie hum going, almost all the time – interrupted only by the distraction of his favorite grains – and then the humming would start again. I'd witnessed the hum before, when their brother Rev was passing. I put my arm around his neck and asked him if he missed Win as much as I did. I swear his eyes began to mist over. We showed him a large canvas of Winston and his cycle handlebar ears curved over, as he focused on the photo. I knew he recognized him.

Nowadays, his 400lb self can be mostly seen on the deck, sometimes blocking the entire entrance way, so the dogs have to alert me to move him if they need to pass by. It is quite the strangest thing. My husband never constructed the deck for a llama creature's weight, so some reinforcements will be necessary in the coming months. When we open the sliding door to the house, Harold will peek in and stand stock still with fascination. I'm sure, one day, he will be in the family room, stretched out on the cool wooden floor with the pups. I know my llama shearer would tell me this is not regular llama behavior; but I couldn't care less how irregular he is in the llama world. I love it and I'm certain it helps me deal with loss. I can groom Harold now, as well as his brother Max, who used to be such a scaredy-cat. They seem to quite like it. Brother Sam will also feed out of the hand now. Things at Solace have changed for sure.

My sister Rosie used to tell me how much she loved butterflies. "Yeah, but they live for such a short time!" I said to her once. "Yes, sister, that's the whole point. They are really beautiful, and they live short lives. Enjoy them while they are here! All about the quality, not the quantity!" And, of course, at the time – duh – I knew she was talking about more than just butterflies. She was quite the butterfly herself throughout her pretty short life. My Secret Garden has become a plethora of magic since Rosie passed. I built the Rosie boat in her memory – she loved boats, she loved water; I needed a memorial site for her close to me and so the boat was built. I found the abandoned wreck on my Mum's beach in Moss Landing, where we had scattered her ashes. I found the memorial on the day that Rosie was transitioning, so it was all perfect. I lay beautiful things in front of the old piece of boat, including sea glass and stones from beaches I loved, dragon fly images, a Sir Win White Horseshoe, a mermaid and much more. When I talk to my turtles and feed them in the mornings, I am often reminded of what a special place my Secret Garden is, as the butterflies flitter by, the humming birds dive and stun with their glorious array of colors and the dragonflies whoosh through your viewshed, sometimes with their babies in tow. Ever seen a baby dragonfly? It is the most astounding tiny slip of metallic colors you have ever seen. The mama is a green and blue beauty – she likes to come and swim with me, as my sister would – her babies stay in the sanctuary of the Secret Garden and the stalks of the long grasses. I can't wait to watch them grow up. They say that the dragonfly is a messenger from another realm, and I certainly believe that to be true. Dragonflies were very special to my sister and me. Equally, she knew they'd be very precious to me after she'd passed.

When I was in England, my friend and I went night swimming in the sea. The Mama Cormorant – my mother's spirit creature – was nesting above us in the basket of a metal groin, as we swam beneath her. I told my friend my mother would never let us swim without her watching us; no matter that we were good swimmers. Sometimes this meant hours of her time, perched on the beach just watching. I felt the same thing about the cormorant. She would have been watching especially cautiously at night. I felt her presence. I called out her name.

When Winston passed, I saw his spirit animal evolve as the elegant white doves that frequent our place – they eat and drink and nest and live peacefully in our trees, lots of them. This gift means that I see him all the time – exactly as I need to. If there are two doves together, then he is with his beloved Abbey Rhode – our gentle brown mare – who passed a few years ago and whose passing made me a believer in the fact that animals do grieve and, boy, he did, for 2 whole weeks.

"Good morning, Sir Winston White Bird!" I chirp as I go out of a morning. "Morning Bud!" I say as the dragonfly greets me at the gates to my secret garden. "Mum!" I see the cormorant swooping over the Pacific on her way to grab breakfast. And who will tell me I am wrong, or at least insane. My perception of the world and my loss is eased by seeing my beloveds in the bodies of other things, since I can't see them in person. They live at my home we call Solace and this all serves to provide me with immense comfort.

(2019)

Making good memories

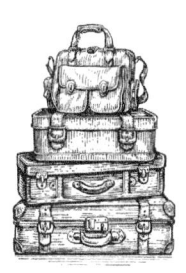

I hate the 4th of July, America's birthday, Independence Day and all that. There I've said it. I even said it out loud, as I hummed, alternatively, *Star Spangled Banner* and *We are the Champions*. Then a war-time mortar comes flying over my head and I scream and duck for cover, army-crawling towards the house in retreat.

I'm not even kidding. It has been about 3 weeks now of insanely violent and obnoxiously invasive noise – firecrackers, bombs, illegal this and that – who knows what all has been lighting up the local streets and frightening the pets to pieces, leaving piles of scummy trash everywhere and hearts that are still missing a beat. There are so many lost and found animals posted recently that it makes me sick to my stomach. If I did not keep my animals inside during this invasion of my privacy, they would, for sure, break down the doors to get in. I've even had one of my dogs break out through a barbed wire fence one holiday season and run for the hills. Luckily some kind soul found him, and he was chipped, or he'd still be running.

Is this acceptable? I mean really. Who enjoys all that white noise, that violation of our Constitution? Even selling the so-called safe and sane fireworks does not seemingly slow the public's passion for the illegal stuff. The other night, my neighbors' dogs busted out of their yard and came to my house, waking all of us. My dogs were already going crazy, the skies were booming; and it sounded as if we really were in the middle of a war zone. I understand that our law enforcement has a heck of a time trying to track down the violators, but what about the neighbors of the obnoxious? Why don't they report them? When did we become such an apathetic nation?

Years ago, I was proud of the 4th of July and all she stood for. I became an American Citizen right before the 4th, and I wore my colors proudly. I even got to lead the group in the Pledge of Allegiance with my mother's sparkly Old Glory hat perched firmly on my head and I thought it would be forever a favorite and symbolic holiday. But now, I cannot wait for it to be over. Even if we were not in the middle of a pandemic, I would never leave my house, because of my animals' fears and my own fear that my house might burn down. We eat our hamburgers in acknowledgment of America's birthday and then run inside, turn up the television and hope for the best.

Friends of mine leave town with all their animals and head for the middle of nowhere, as far from humanity as they can get. I would do that too, if transporting my llamas and the rest of them were not quite so tricky. Plus, you've got the whole house burning down thing. Fireworks in high summer with all our dry brush and fire volatility? Ludicrous at best.

On the 5th of July, we breathe a sigh of relief. Though tired from a sleepless night trying to comfort our traumatized pups, we are intact. The house is still standing, and all my fur babies are present and accounted for, if suffering from a dose of PTSD. For many others, that is not the case. Piles of toxic waste line our residential streets in town and there are notices everywhere for missing pups. I can only imagine how scared they are out there alone in the wilderness. Makes me sick that America's birthday has become the holiday to despise, the recapturing of war-time experience that no one should have to visit and the dumping ground for all the fools who like to scare others, especially the animals that cannot protect themselves, not to mention the Veterans who suffer with post war stress and, in serving their country, so did not earn that measure of disrespect. Friends of mine tell me their special needs children have to be specially prepared with earphones and comfort blankets in order to get through these days, the celebration of America's birthday that has become such a tiresome and unenjoyable mess.

On another note, today would have been my sister Rosie's wedding anniversary. She and her beloved husband Ali were only married for a wonderfully sweet 4 years, before she left us; but their time together was so precious it covered decades. Knowing time is short can make it the most precious ever. They traveled the world – Spain, Venice, Kenya, Kilimanjaro and all over. They made sure all the memories were lasting, as their marriage could not be. When you are thinking about making memories for your loved ones, why not veer towards the precious and constructive. How about you light pretty sparklers with your children, BBQ some burgers, talk about the reason for the holiday and not terrify them with the explosions and cracks? Life really is too short for all that chaos and mayhem. Make good memories that will not only make you and yours happy, but also everyone else in your neighborhood.

(2019)

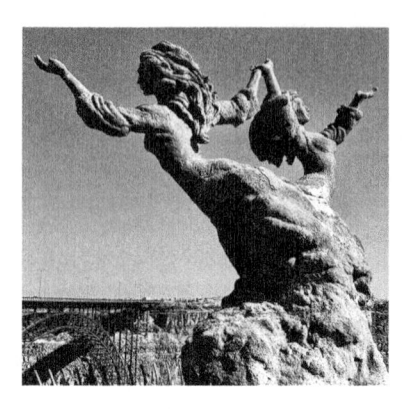

My big birthday

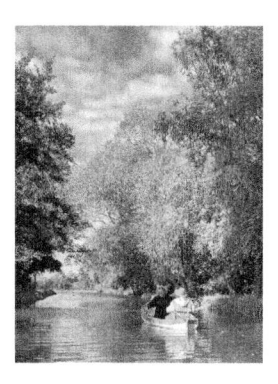

It was likely about half a century since I had even paused at the bend of that place. It was created as a playground in the 1920's by Ogilvie, a Scottish barrister, this watery wonderland boating lake, which was inspired by his friend JM Barrie's Peter Pan. The 60-acre lake – allegedly dug out by hand – is a fantasy land of little creeks and waterways with *islands* (a relative term) where you can rest your rowing boat that boast names like Wendy's Home, Pirate's Lair and the Blue Lagoon.

We just called it the Thorpeness Meare, (not a familiar American term, I'm sure) and, as kids, our parents would drop us off so that we could row in 2 feet of water to our heart's delight and play Swallows and Amazons or pirates and torment the boys. We had loved the freedom this afforded our young selves with huge imaginations and large appetites for mischief. It was only a skip from the beach, but truly miles away.

Thorpeness has always been a bit of a strange burg, just down the road from Aldeburgh in Suffolk where I was born but sporting largely anonymous white clapboard houses with black crisscrossed beams throughout, a tiny village store, a country club and this fantasy lake. It was never considered a real place to live in our minds and we had no friends there. It was almost as if Peter Pan himself resided there, along with a host of other imaginary characters.

"What do you want to do for your 60th birthday?" Friends were gathering in Aldeburgh in various cottages, and we surely needed to do something to mark the day the 'baby' of the group turned a big number, so a trip to the Meare was sprung upon the unsuspecting visitors, most of whom had last visited the lake decades before. Since my oldest friend and I were working on the story of our childhood in Aldeburgh together, it seemed apt that we should revisit the Meare, one of the chapters in our story.

I was delighted to see that the boats were literally the same ones from our childhood – old wooden rowing boats painted in all colors of the rainbow and named Rose Bud, Lizzie, Sally, Mavis … they were just as rocky to get in as they ever were and equally uncomfortable with wooden board seats and no cushions.

There were 3 boats and 2 dogs that took off from the side this Sunday and rowed steady-ish through the mossy water towards the fantasy land, howling with laughter. I'm not sure exactly what we were expecting, but nothing in those watery lands had changed. The passing of time had been suspended in this place. Even the marauding swans were just as rude as they were 50 years ago, one leaning his hawky beak into our boat and scaring me silly. Even the *islands* were the same, but we didn't feel the need to jump out of the boats this go-around, lest we rock the proverbial boat too much and end up with cell phones in the water and ruined shoes. I don't remember ever caring about that years ago and we never had electronics on board in any case.

"I see a snake!" someone yelled and, sure enough, there were water snakes in the mossy waters – quite the eco system, I'm sure, for all the swans, geese, ducks and apparently snakes. The sunshine was glorious and fantastic shots were captured of my special day with blue skies, white swans and green mossy lake in the background.

After our boating expedition, it was time for more cake. One chocolate cake had already been consumed, so it was undoubtedly time for another that my very busy friend had somehow found the time to bake before she came down for birthday weekend. Oh, and a cheesecake that another friend had bought – plus the case of lovely wines and bubblies that father had sent over for another friend to bring with. This celebrating stuff is heavy on the waistline, but certainly light on the heart.

Following boating and cake part 2, it was time for champagne. Then, with ourselves over full of birthday lusciousness, the conversation turned to more serious topics that we should ponder when we are of a certain age. Living trusts, wills, how much money we won't be leaving to our children, poor health and the super tricky subjects of who is in the unfortunate position of an adjustable mortgage that will be resetting next year. These were sobering convos that led us back around to a little more wine, certainly more cake and further reminders of the fragility of life.

The following day I was a bit under the weather with the snuffles and a sore throat – perhaps the result of too much excess over the previous days, too many late nights and the extra gift of a friend who came to visit with a cough. All further plans were immediately canceled, and the 60-year-old self was put to bed with Lemsip, hot tea and her book. After some extra hours of sleep, she was nearly back to normal, save the sore throat, and able to bask a little on the beach which was superbly sunny and kind.

Sometimes it's fun to go backwards in life and forget a bit about adulting, mortgages and living trusts. On occasion, it's freeing to go boating and have a laugh, drink champagne and too much cake. We did all of that this weekend and, I'm proud to say, we survived, and no one fell in the water.

(2023)

October is a funny old month!

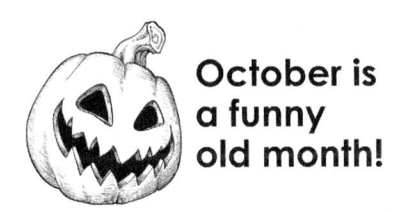

October is a funny old month. Some days are hot as summer, with stilled winds and an icy bite to the early mornings and evenings. November can be more of the same, yet the time of year is marked by the turn of the vines – the rich colors bending from yellows and greens to dark reds and near black hues. I love this time of year, though my body struggles with the changing temperatures and oftentimes fights a cold through the transition of the seasons.

As I drove across the valley, I was stunned by the array of autumnal colors – the swathes of yellow and green, then the fall vines telling us about the time of the year, fruit flies hanging onto the last drips of nectar. Halloween is just a memory of rotting pumpkins and seasonal décor leaning towards Thanksgiving, one of the most civilized dates on the American calendar. As I crossed the green bridge onto Arroyo Seco Road and saw the whisper of the river still running, I felt overcome with gratitude for the place we call home, the beauty of the hills and fields, the blessing of the fresh airs. We really do live in one of the most beautiful places on earth.

And here we are a skip away from Thanksgiving. I recall my early experiences of Thanksgiving – the strange mixes of fruit and jelly on a plate with turkey and sweet potato. I may not have understood the combination of flavors, but I learned to accept them in my palate and enjoy the meaning of the season.

Our childhood memoir

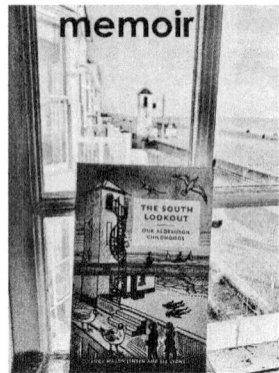

My friend and I have been writing the story of our shared childhood. I say *my friend* meaning my oldest friend in the whole world. The story goes that she fell into the boating pond in my hometown (all of 2 feet deep) when we were both about 4, my mother fished her out and, from there, our families became firm friends. Her parents then went on to, thoughtfully, purchase a house next to ours in this seaside town and from there a forever friendship between us flourished.

Every weekend and holiday, we would be headed to our homes by the coast from our homes in the country or city. She was always the last to show up and I would wait impatiently for her to arrive on the Friday night. As soon as I heard the car doors bang next door, I was out of our front door at Number 39 – no matter the time – and into her house at Number 43 and then we were off out again. Our homes were situated on a parallel street to the seafront that led to the beach and then the sea – in a small town that had one way in and one way out – still does. The next street over was the high street with our favorite shops. From the chip shop to the sweetie shop, toy shop and bookshop; that was our playground and our parents never worried about us. We came and went as we pleased. It was a blissful existence. Even then we knew how very lucky we were.

It has been so fun and such a brain exercise to dig back 56 years ago or so, and then crawl slowly forwards in our quest to put some kind of an interesting 1970's journal together of our formative years in our beloved coastal town. During my last trip there, we sat at the kitchen table of my old cottage (that we managed to rent through Air B n B no less) and scratched away at the surface of our shared memories over a glass of wine or three. So interesting how different recollections and varied interpretations emerge after all this time with much common ground in-between.

Both of my friends' parents and my own mother and sister are now gone, but it has been so delightful bringing them back to life, as it were, through photos and shared memory banks. We have used my father as an enormous resource in the process. Though up there in years, he boasts a still razor-sharp memory and an enormous recollection of the history of the time and memory of where and when, historian that he is. We are inserting into our story his recollections too, since this was such a very two-family tale – it's not just about she and I at all. Actually, many more than two families – truth be told – we were the King Street Gang – a minimum of 4 houses, adults and kids, with other friends around the periphery and up the town – that enjoyed this marvelous life parallel to the sea front and a skip from the beach and sea that we loved so much.

No matter where I have lived in the world, this seaside town of Aldeburgh has always been my home. It has been the most consistent geographic landmark of my existence, even though I haven't lived there permanently since I was a small child.

Recreating our childhoods and immersing ourselves with our family members now departed from this planet has been a cathartic endeavor for both of us. We have dug deep for photos and info, laughed hard at some of the images and letters we found stamped by time (remember those?) and tried to create a nice mixture of text and image for our audience.

Our childhood town is a very well-known burg for art and music and has been for years. Many famous people have resided and/or worked within its boundaries, so we are in good company with our manuscript to be. I am fortunate that my old mucker Lizzie is a graphic designer par excellence and can throw together a book with images like no one's business (see our last shared project *The Soup Diaries*, styling and layout entirely her work!) We are hopeful that the bookshop of our youth will be happy to sell our book within its hallowed walls, (our mothers both had charge accounts there for years that Lizzie and I used the heck out of! Has to count for something!) And it will be exciting to share our tome with our many family and friends who also love our town alongside us. But more than that, it is about putting all the memories in one place, collecting the 1970's technicolor photo images, looking at my mother's large body of work (pen and ink drawings and oil paintings) from the place and giving a nod to her incredible talent and love for our town, preserving all of it for generations to come.

Our project has forced me to go through photos and be selective. No more clumps of sticky snapshots in a placcy box. We need to extract, scan and insert for posterity. Sometimes even have them beautifully framed!

I recently also purchased a bench with a plaque for us all on the sea front in our town and in the neighborhood of all our old houses. At the ripe old age of 6 decades on the planet, I feel as if it's past time to braid together lots of old threads and push the projects in my brain to print, as it were.

As a writer, you are never done. Though I sometimes question why I do this at all. I will never make a living at it – let's face it – but it does serve a purpose to fill a void inside myself, a need to tell the stories that may matter to some in my circle who may care, especially once I'm gone. I have a few other stories inside me that must be told before I leave our planet, so self-motivation is a good thing and that's something I'm not lacking. As my baby sister would fondly say …'better get my sh*t together!'

For right now, my old friend Lizzie and I are hoping to get this baby to bed by the holidays, or before she goes on her crazy round -the-world sailing expedition at the very least. She has oceans to sail, and I have other books to write. I'll let you know when our shared project has been safely birthed.

(2023)

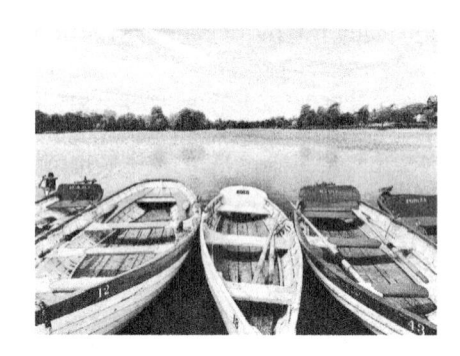

Passion

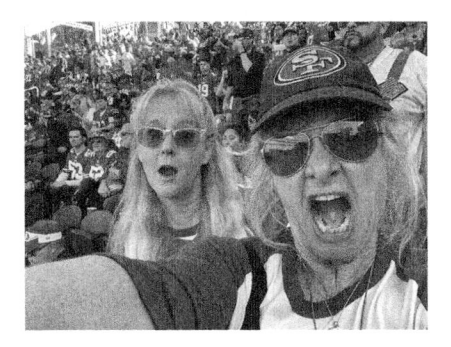

Why do you like it so much? He asked. You could ask a lot of people that same question and they wouldn't be stumped the way I was. I thought back to the beginning of the passion, the birth of my new hobby. My friend was picking me up to take me to a game – a new experience indeed. I knew the color of the team, but I was dressed in the exact opposite – in fact the other team's colors – that just about ensured I wouldn't be attending the game that day. I had no clue, obviously, what the color and support theme was all about. I recall a lot of hoopla on my first adventure and thinking how attractive the players looked in their uniforms. I didn't have any idea what was going on, but that didn't seem to matter. There was a lot of noise, banter, color, music and enthusiasm going on and I really liked that. From there I purchased the book *Football for Dummies*. I wanted to learn a little more about this captivating sport where the young men dressed to kill, and everyone else seemed really enthused. Next a hat was purchased and then my own shirt or two in the appropriate colors.

Fortunately, my son patiently explained some of the fundamental rules of the game. When he was a young high schooler, I had attended a few of his games with the *Watsonville Wild Catz* and appreciated nothing about the game except for the hot chocolate at the concession stands and the relative brevity of the game. Was I now becoming a bit of a fan? What is all this business about first down, second down, interception, snap? There was a whole new language to learn; but the more I learned, the more I enjoyed this delightful escape from regular life. I could attend a game, whether in my living room or, blissfully, at the stadium itself and Lucy-Responsible-Working-Person had, all of a sudden, left the building. She was yelling and hollering with the fans out there, all cheering on their side. There is something very equalizing about sport. It didn't matter that some of the fans have tattoos over their eyeballs and I was pretty freshly off the boat from Blighty. The football fan base is a very unifying thing. The guy in the grocery store asks me about the upcoming prospects when he eyes my hat and I eye his. "What do you think? We will probably clinch this one, huh?" "Yes, we should." "We should never have won last week," we chuckle. "Oh no, that was a train wreck!" … and so, the banter goes on. A conversation that would never have started over the avocados and lettuce in the corner market – unless we were both on the same team. And I like that about football, I really do. There isn't the bullying mantra that I have witnessed in other sports. There's no caging the fans if they are on the other side. People all sit together with different colors and cheers and that is all part of the game. Pity an East Coast fan who attends a 49er game amidst a sea of red, but they are welcome to cheer along their team just as we are. And there's the *We* again – it's the best kind of group to belong to – a club where everyone loves the same thing and feels really positive and enthusiastic about something in their lives. Let's face it – many folks experience a lot of pressure and division in their daily existence – football is the great equalizer; the place where you can just relax, have fun and forget about all your worries. It's a place of euphoria, truthfully. From the game day excitement, (driving to the game with lots of ardent fans doing the same thing), or taking the train, to entering the stadium, visiting the concessions and the Pro Shop, settling in your seats, watching the players warm up and often famed alumni from the game showing up and giving the crowd a rise, then there is the spectacle of the national anthem, the military colors, often a fly over and some pomp and circumstance. The game is not too long and not too short. Often, we win the ones we shouldn't and lose the ones we shouldn't. Frequently, the craziest things happen to turn a game around and the crowd oohs and aahs with excitement. People leap out of their seats as, out of nowhere, a touchdown is achieved, and the masses go wild. Often an interception happens to turn the tide of the game. It is all very exciting and unexpected – a bit like life itself.

Football is a passion and a pastime. I hate to miss a game and, if I do, I record it to watch later and try to avoid any social media in the meantime, where there might be mention of who won. I treasure my football time. I know all the players and the injury statuses; I enjoy watching the locker room postmortem and the Monday morning quarterback analyses of what happened.

It is good to have passions and I have many. From reading and writing and ranching to animal welfare and … well football. It's all positive good fun and I would highly recommend it to someone looking for some passion and color in their lives. It doesn't have to be football, it could be cycling, basketball or any pursuit that takes you out of yourself and your daily life. When I am at a football game, I feel young, free and unfettered. I have no cares in the world; I'm just buoyant with the simple joys of the day ahead. I do not like to lose – who does – but at least I don't cry like the guy in front of me. I will accept the result of a fair match, as we all must, and look forward to a better result next time. Football is like life – it's not always pretty, but there are some great views along the way.

Dad, does that explain it a bit?

(2021)

Regrets

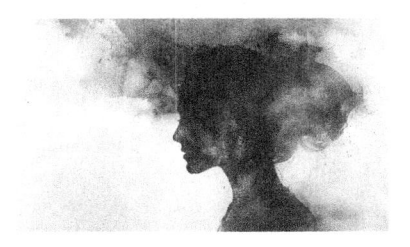

'Regrets … I have a few… ..'

As old as I am now, I can look back and honestly say that most of my regrets are for things I didn't do, say or ask – before it was too late to do anything about it. Nowadays, I live with that in my rear-view mirror. I'm cautious about turning down an invitation or adventure, lest it adds to my regret pile. I don't want to miss out on anything that is important to my people – whether it be weddings, funerals, or even just a last chance to make it right. Maybe that is why I have become the *Event Queen* in my house. If something comes up that I can book, I don't want to miss it. In place of gifts, I give an experience. I gave my friend kayaking on the Pacific – a bucket list item for her – my daughter tickets to see various musicians she coveted from Rihanna and Adele to Tim McGraw and beyond. I'm always on the look-out for a musician I have wanted to see, a play I've been waiting to watch, a game I cannot stand to miss! This can be quite an expensive habit, as I'm sure you can appreciate. It's a habit my sister Rosie started years ago, and I don't think I will be able to ever quit it; it's so much fun.

Her: 'Mum, we haven't been to a game all season!"

Me: 'Oh, do you want tickets for Christmas?"

Her: 'OMG, Mum, yesssss!"

And there with a quick visit to Stubhub, I'm all done with Christmas for her and her boyfriend. Not a scrap of wrapping paper or mailing bag in sight. It's a priceless gift that takes up residency in the memory bank. It's a gift, as they say, that keeps on giving, since I've noticed my daughter adopting the same habit. A nice thing to hand down! I can remember every concert I have been to in my life – from the Stones, Bowie, Madonna, Madness, Eric Clapton, Coldplay, Willie Nelson and more, lest I bore those of you not fans of the concert life. And then there are the multitudes of plays I have attended, far too many to list, but I could if I wanted.

The regrets are also harshly etched on the memory bank. I should and could have gone and visited a very old friend before she died. I didn't make the trip. I wish I had. My baby sister's wedding … shame on me, never will quite get over that one. I had just seen her in England the month before and couldn't see my way to making the long trip from the US to Turkey so soon. At her wedding, she was re-diagnosed with bone cancer/stage 4, and I wasn't there. "I really thought you'd surprise me, sis," she noted after the fact. Ouch, that hurt. I should have made the trip. There are no excuses for that, except that there are – there is only so much money to go around, and I do have to work. International travel is expensive, I live so very far away.... I have bills to pay, jobs to do … no, I know. There is NO excuse not to attend your sister's wedding. She came to both of yours. Regret is a beast that can gnaw away at you, no matter how much time passes. Then there was the time I thought I really shouldn't make the trip; it seemed really long and decadent; but I wanted to go so badly, I just made it happen. My baby sis and all her closest friends were meeting up in Istanbul for Valentine's weekend. She invited me to come, and I couldn't think of reasons I should go, except I wanted to. So, I went. What an amazing weekend for the memory banks. We walked, ate, visited the sights of the city, laughed so much, danced on a boat and more …plus we took lots and lots of photos and videos. That's another thing; when you document your special times, then you can enjoy it over and over again. This past weekend was the anniversary of that trip, and I was able to revisit all the amazing things we did in photographic form all over again. "Thanks for the memories!" said one of the weekenders. "Oh, such precious memories!" said another. No one can take those images out of your memory bank, no matter what. They are beautifully cluttered up in there along with the regrets and, hopefully, they soften up those regrets a little, as they should. Because, after all, you can do nothing with the darned regret issue, but wish it were otherwise.

So, take a leaf out of my book and buy the experiences, make sure you go out and make the memories and try to avoid any regret. When I'm an old lady – if I live that long – I plan to look back on my amazing life with as few regrets as I can muster.

(2020)

Rocket Man

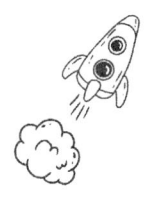

It had been a long time coming. Our newsie friend moved from California a few decades back and had been asking us to come and visit for the longest time. There was always a reason we couldn't make it. Why couldn't we make it? Time whizzes past us, doesn't she; positively gallops, the older you get.

"Elton John is coming to Arkansas!" She tells us. "It's his farewell tour. You need to come!" Well, now we had no reason to find a reason we couldn't go. I jumped on the site to try and buy tickets. The tickets were a *little* high, but what's high when a legend is doing his final trip around the world. We booked our airline tickets and began to mark the calendars and look forward to the new adventure. "You always need dates in the diary," my friends and I often remind each other.

Then along came our uninvited guest Madame Covid and everything got pushed down to the dark ditches of living. Flights and concerts were all postponed. We were not going to see the legend; we were not going anywhere. 2020 sat heavy on the hearts and shoulders of all of us, like a complete fun sucker.

Then The Legend needed a surgery, and we collectively held our breath all over again. Oh no, not another cancellation! We had already pushed our plan into the next year and tomorrow is never guaranteed, is it. I want to do everything I ever wanted in my life, until I can no more. Can't fester any regrets when I'm an old lady in my chair. We went ahead and booked our travel for the rescheduled dates and penciled it – only pencil, mind – into our calendars for early the following year. "Heal well, old friend!" we said quietly to the interiors of our own walls. I love to see legends. There is something so grounding and marvelous about the planned and gracious exit of a fabulous and impressive career, (though I did see the Rolling Stones in Leeds in 1982 and wondered, at the time, if that was going to be their last tour. Ha!)

Then the 3rd triangle of our party was not going to be able to make it. Though our uninvited guest Madame Covid seemed to be now moderately cooperating with the travel plans of the world, we were losing a corner of our triangle. Life had got in the way, and she wasn't going to be able to make the party. We were gutted. Dang, if it wasn't one thing it was another. I hate it when that happens. Were we going to make it? Was the party ever going to happen? Was the writing on the proverbial wall that we finally had to dump the whole brilliant idea down the drain of blank-blank happens?

Tomorrow Is Not Promised

I didn't even want to tell anyone what the plan was and had been for two years now. That might make the scheme somehow permanently evaporate, as have so many along the road of annihilated plans in recent times. "Will he be there, will he not?" There were whispers along the corridors of the adventurous that he wasn't feeling well. Heck. I get a text. "He has covid!" No!!! "He has canceled Dallas!" Well, now. I wasn't canceling my flight or my plans this time. I was just going to go and enjoy regardless. My friend had taken days off and we would have fun. "You're leaving again?" my daughter seemed surprised. I didn't have the energy to explain the whole story to her.

Right up until the day of, we did not know for sure if we would be attending the 'Farewell Yellow Brick Road' grand finale concert of Sir Elton John in Little Rock. Apparently, the Dallas concert – the previous stop on the tour – had been canceled just a few hours before showtime, so we kept nervously checking our messages and email. At about 4pm, we decided the show would be going on and we primped a little and headed out for the concert hall – via the Irish Pub, as you do. Gotta get a little sauced up for a mega event such as this. To our surprise and delight, glam rock came out that day in downtown Little Rock. From the feathers and sequins to the white platform boots and gold sparkly trousers, we were back in the 1970's and there was going to be a show. And boy did he show up! At 74 years old, he absolutely killed it. There were young and old at the party, the able-bodied and the infirm. He sang through many of his considerable repertoire over the course of two plus hours, pausing only to chat to the crowd or sip on his water. It seemed as if he enjoyed it as much as we did, also acknowledging exactly how many days it had been since we were supposed to have been together; and now we were. I felt quite teary at times, finally getting to see the Legend, against the odds, live on stage. He might not be dancing on the piano in his platforms anymore, but he performed like an absolute king and boasted a lovely, sweet humbleness that sang through his performance. As he was elevated up and into the scenery after the last encore, in his robe and slippers no less, we all had such a good laugh at this marvelous man who had given so much not only to the world of music, but also to humanity at large. His work with the AIDS foundation and his ongoing efforts to push for acceptance of gays and gay marriage in the world have pushed him up to the levels of way beyond a composer and musician, but to a historic level of complete hero.

For those of you who couldn't make the final concert tour, I urge you to read his incredible biography "Rocket Man' and also see the film. You'll be glad you did.

Not only did we finally accomplish our goals that had seemed lost in the large slice of life spent with Madame Covid, but I got to know a whole new State and I love that. We toured the Clinton Library – remarkable – visited the school of the Arkansas 9 – sobering – and soaked in the cuisine and the ambiance of the deep south everywhere we went – from the Cotton Shed to the Cracker Barrel and beyond.

Thanks must go out to Susan, my hostess and friend of 30 plus years. What a fabulous time we had; most certainly opening the gateway to many more epic times and laughs galore.

And thank you, Rocket Man, for all the music and all the years. Go raise those beautiful children with your beautiful husband. Be happy. I think you finally are.

(PS I went to see Rocket Man again in California later in the year. What a lucky girl!)

(2022)

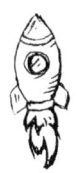

Take care of yourself

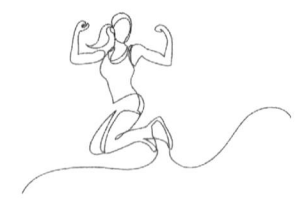

"Take care of yourself!" They rant. "Diet and exercise, exercise and diet." Yes, we all know about that. Some of us consistently live by excellent habits, others less so. I've always loved to swim and walk – that's my idea of exercise – and I used to think I did pretty well with that keeping me upright, until last summer that is.

After my super clumsy, also dumb escapade with a horse and an air-flying corral board that knocked me out and took me to the ground, my knee was pretty smashed up. I acknowledge that you are likely to get regularly beat up when you do daily ranch work. I'm always boasting a few bruises and scrapes here and there; but this injury was a little different. "You didn't even think of going to see the doc?" (Well, no, I never do!) People seemed surprised. I just expect wounds to heal and swellings to disappear. Always have. Until they don't.

We are onto the 9th month of me talking boringly about my messed-up knee and the forever and a day it is taking to heal. Once the gash itself closed up, the wounded area was numb for quite some time and the limp seemed to just get worse. I did stretches, I got massages. I was digging deep into the 'I'm not going to the doc' toolbox that I mostly carry under my arm.

"You need to get that seen to, Lu, before it gets chronic," father noted. "Gosh, your walking is much worse than it was the last time," sister sternly chided me when I admitted that I had done absolutely nothing about it since my last visit.

And then when we went out walking, the change was marked. I had a hard time keeping up with my little sister, where previously my gait had always been strong and swift. It was well past time to do something mature to stop the decline.

I went to see the doc and he was markedly surprised that I had been doing the wounded warrior thing for several months. He sent me for x-rays and gave me some anti-inflamms – also told me to get my limpy self to the physiotherapist. He thought that I had tendonitis in the knee, plus some stubborn scar tissue that wasn't allowing the knee to properly heal.

I had never been to physio before, and it was quite the work out. From balls to bands to stretchy machines and ankle torture, not to mention the stationary bike and shock machine, I realized that this was a whole different world outside of my few lame leg stretches and hoping for the best that hadn't really worked out for me. This was the world of fix-it, if not swiftly, at least eventually.

"Do you think I can avoid surgery?" I asked meekly of the physio, eyes in the doggy downwards position. "I think so," he said. "But you are going to have to work really hard." And then it was onto the enthusiastic purchase of yoga mats and balls to work the knee and leg, I downloaded the app for daily exercises and vowed to bounce back stronger than ever with my gimpy knee fixed and an athletic resolve to not be stupid like that ever again. I even purchased husband his own yoga mat and we resolved to try and improve our levels of fitness together. After all, I am going to be 60 this year and my athleticism and suppleness will not take care of themselves.

We are a month into my new physio routine, and it is quite time-consuming trying to fit the two sessions in every week, but I am determined to emerge victorious. Already my knee seems to be less stiff and achy (I also go to the massage therapist as often as possible for some further work on the area.) I am investing a boat load of mullah into remedying this situation (my health insurance covers neither physio nor massage by the way ...) Though I still suffer with an aching leg and foot on the dodgy side, especially at night, I am already walking less like someone who needs an immediate hip or knee replacement and more like the girl I used to know.

I'm hoping, when I see father and sister next month, they will be very happy with my improved physical prowess, and I will be able to walk the doggy with sister like I used to. Disability is not a joke, people, and it creeps up on you like a slow and persistent plague when you are super busy doing other things.

A lesson to anyone who will listen. If you do something stupid to yourself, go and get it checked out by a medical professional and then follow the doc's orders. Do not be a ranch warrior like me and live to regret your stubborn self months down the road, when your injury is no longer affecting just the joint itself, but your entire body, not to mention your life.

And then this week, what do I go and do? I slide on a muddy stable mat, land on my back and my wrist and my wrist quickly swells up like a ball. "Ice it, mother, right now!" my nurse daughter tells me. And I immediately do. In fact, we have an ice pack in our freezer ready to go for incidents like that. Though it was sore the next day, it was headed on its way down to being a normal wrist again and I felt as if I had finally learned something about self-care and response time.

Though I still have a ways to go until I am no longer under doc's orders, and I do wonder what the night throbs are in the leg and foot, I feel so much better about my prognosis than I did a month ago. I have been putting in the work and I now think I shall be striding out unaided for years to come. If you are a stubborn wench like me, heed my cautionary tale. I am no longer 15 years-old and my old bits no longer fix themselves. Be less like me and more like a mature person who wants to preserve their mobility for as long as possible.

(2023)

The Best Made Plans

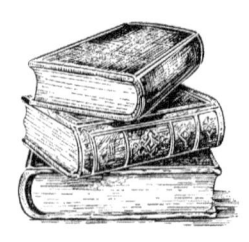

The best made plans, as they say, can get really messed up. It was late fall 2019 and I was trying to finish up my corrections for my book manuscript. These days, to be current, you need to publish on Kindle and paper, even though golden oldies like myself always prefer the paper version, something you can touch and physically turn the pages. I still like to read a regular newspaper for crying out loud; I'm what they call *tactile* (or old-fashioned, if you like)!

I got myself in a bit of a pickle with the fact that, in this modern world, you also need to edit two separate sets of corrections for the Kindle format and the *regular* one. Not being, perhaps, the sharpest tool in the shed, I started working on the Kindle corrections first. Why I did that still concerns me as a self-considered fairly intelligent human. I was planning on having actual book copies ready for the holidays, I was intending to deliver glossy-covered tomes to my nearest and dearest when I went to England for Christmas. Can't wrap up a Kindle story, now can you? My father was getting impatient – this baby had really taken far too long to deliver; finally, I sent the now-edited Kindle version to him for the bargain basement price of $2.99. "No, Lu," he said by way of thanks. "I want the hard copy." Well, phooey.

I rushed the corrections through on the paper manuscript version, imagining that they would be awaiting my return in January and then I could plan my signings and launch my book properly in the New Year. Hadn't really made it in time for the holiday rush, but oh well. Character is fate, as they say. January would be better for book signings anyway, when folks didn't have so much to do and could enjoy, perhaps, a little chunk of local creativity.

I received my hard copy in the mail. Glossy and gorgeous on the outside, I was really very proud. It had taken me such a very long time to finish. I flicked through the stories inside. "Oh no! Something had gone wrong with the pagination; there were errors I didn't catch. Granny's words *More haste less speed* rushed through my brain. Had I taken my time and not been in such a beastly hurry, this would not be happening.

"Don't buy it," I told my friends. It's on Amazon all over the world, but don't buy it. I was mortified. I made my dad promise he wouldn't buy it either, because it was such a horrible mess, I would never live it down.

When I got back to the US, I worked staunchly on my corrections. Gosh I was so sick of the darn thing. You forget that when you are planning a fresh writing enterprise. You forget how tedious the editing is, the proofing, blah blah, so tiresome. But if you can't afford an editor, *needs must* … another of my blessed granny's sayings. I trolled through the manuscript and resubmitted for the changes. I asked my friend in England if she could check that the Amazon.co.uk site had now got the edited version. I waited. She ordered her copy and confirmed that they had. I sent a copy over to my father and sister. No comments meant that they must have reasonably enjoyed the book; or perhaps it was still sitting on the coffee table, waiting for someone to care less.

Anyhow, the book is finally done, and I order 100 copies. I scheduled some book signings, start marketing the signings and then along comes Corona. "You have got to be kidding me!" What is it with my timing these days? Just as well my signing for next week cannot happen – I just received a message from Amazon that my print job has been delayed and they will notify me when delivery can occur.

I do hope that spring will be kinder to me and my elusive third book publication. I look forward to being able to move freely within society, hug whoever I want to and, perhaps, host a nice tea party book signing for my third book. *The Animals Teach Us Everything & Other Short Tails* is, I think, a really a very nice collection of my mostly animal stories from my newspaper columns 2011-2019 and it's illustrated with my own photos. If anyone would like a signed copy, I'll have some coming eventually and I would be glad to mail one to you while we are all on lockdown and needing entertainment.

(2020)

The books that made me

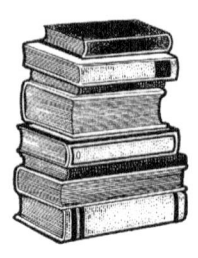

One of my earliest memories was my mother's voice. I was on her lap, and she was reading to me. We were likely in our cottage by the sea with a fire blazing in the hearth. She had a good strong reading voice with superb inflexion and read to me all the time. I loved listening to her. The Beatrix Potter collection was an early firm favorite – with the animal characters so interesting and complex – accompanied by divine illustrations. I still have some of those very worn little books; some of them with my younger sister's crayon graffiti inside, just in case I ever thought something was really mine. I also still have my childhood *Orlando, the Marmalade Cat,* a deliciously imaginative story about an orange cat and his family who live in Owlborough-on-Sea – a play on the little seaside town where I grew up. For forever and a day, Mum gave that book to whoever was having a baby. It was an absolute must-have. Still is.

The classics – *A Little Princess and the Secret Garden* by Frances Hodges Burnett were read so many times by me, that their covers and dog-eared pages were deeply imprinted on my brain. I could only imagine how devastating it would be to be an orphan, alone in the world with no one really wanting you. I do remember how safe and fortunate it made me feel that I had a loving family that would never abandon me in that way. *A Little White Horse* was another beloved novel that began my love of the magic white horse that stays with me to this day. I can still re-read all these books from my formative years, and I am back there in the mind of a young girl.

Books are fundamental to a good education, in my opinion. I read to my girl when she was still in the womb and brought her up as a reader with stories every night before bed. She was not plonked in front of an electronic babysitter; at least, full disclosure; not often. The evening was our time to read together and relax before bed. In grade school, she entered the Countywide Spelling Bee and did very well. Often, I would read the same story over and over to her and then she began to want to read to me. *The Story of Ping, You are not my mother, Peep-Po, Junie-B Jones* … the list goes on and on. One summer I challenged her to read 100 books from the library and she did. I do believe her prize was a large soft dog. To this day, she is a most excellent speller. I'm working on my granddaughter also being a phenomenal reader. She loves the late-night cuddle and story time as well; the time that you just devote to her without outside influence or noise or banter. It is so important that we give that time to the growing young minds. When Madison Rose last stayed with us, *Are you my mother* had to be read 3 times in a row. She would giggle a lot. "Read it again," she'd say. "Read it again." And I would.

My sister Rosie tried to wean me on to the Kindle. I hear her voice now. "Gotta be done, sis. Gotta be done!" I tried and I couldn't do it. There's something so comforting about an actual book. I savor the covers, the ability to relax in a bath with a story that is not your life, the luxury of lying in a bed with a book. I just can't experience those feelings with a computer, however book-sized it might be. Those of us who are tactile struggle with electronic everythings and, though understanding the rationale, I never accepted the Kindle, even when I travel. "What are you going to do with all those books?" People ask me. I have books and bookshelves all over my house. I do not know the answer to that. I know that if a book has a family member's handwriting in it, I am unable to part with it. Evelyn Burrows .. 1933 (My grandmother's careful hand, the year my mother was born.) Una Baxter .. 1960 (My mother before she married.) These are all anchors in time, and I prize them. I doubt the next generation – the ones who will inherit my books – will feel the same way about them, though perhaps they might keep the books I wrote myself and inscribed. Whatever, it's a life-long passion I shall take with me to the end.

Read to your children and your grandchildren. Open their eyes to the huge world outside and breed curiosity in their minds. Don't leave it for the classroom, make it a vital part of your every day – a special time that you will regularly share, knowing these are precious minutes you are sharing that can't last forever, but that will imprint important memories that your young ones can equally pass along.

I cannot wait to start reading the *Junie B Jones* series to my granddaughter. I know she will howl with laughter, as my daughter and I did years ago. Fortunately, there are a lot of them in the series. My plan is that she will become an excellent reader and writer just like her auntie and that she will love books just like her grandma. She certainly enjoyed my book *Winston Comes Home* and was impressed that her old Grandma had actually written it. These are gifts that we pass down and we need to make the time to share with one another. Life should never be too busy to sit down with a good book and take a walk someplace else.

On my nightstand, there are piles of books that I never get to; mostly because I am always adding to the pile. There are forever books that I just must keep. Michelle Obama's *Becoming* is there, as is *The Little White Horse* (time for a re-read), *The Mayor of Casterbridge* (last read when I was 15) and the list goes on. I'm currently reading the autobiography of Gavanndra Hodges – *The Consequence of Love* – about a girl who loses her younger sister. Now there's a story and a nod to my baby sister Rosie, now years gone from our planet, but never forgotten and often just the wing of a dragonfly away. I can imagine her laughing at my piles of books. "Oh sis. Just no fixing you, is there?" No, likely not. Keep immersed in the world of books, folks. No matter what else is going on, it's a wonderful place to be.

(2020)

The call of the sea

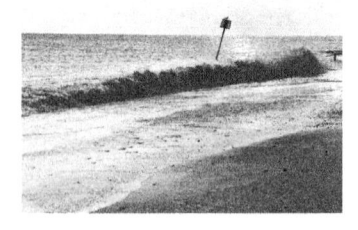

I was born on the East Coast of England and many of my formative years were spent by, in and on the North Sea. To this day I still feel the call of the water. It's so primal. Not just that water, all bodies of water, but especially that one. During the pandemic, I was unable to travel to see my water. In essence, I was banned from visiting my home country for an extended period and it was torture. Having freely crossed the pond, as it were, for over 30 years, I was not able to go. I kept booking flights and they were always canceled. The call of the sea whistled to me from thousands of miles away, echoing my name like a memory I couldn't leave behind.

I visited other bodies of water near my home in California from Pismo to Monterey during those long months of lockdown and forced estrangement from my people. These beaches fed my soul for brief interludes, but I still felt the call from that grey beast overseas – her brownish-grey blue splash onto the shingle, the sparkle of the morning sun, the twinkle of pebble treasures to be found underfoot. My sea, the place where my mother taught me and many others how to swim, where our family spent weekends and summers for years and years; that special place in the world where I can always find my peace.

Finally, September 2021 there was a window of opportunity to return home to my place. Only for 2 days, as it transpired, since my oversea schedule was a hefty one after years away, but I'd take it.

I arrived in town finally and could not wait to get rid of the rental car. I was so beside myself with excitement I parked in a no-parking zone and got myself a rather chunky parking ticket that I cared not a bit about. Without even checking in at the hotel, I scampered down the beach like a child, flinging myself so hard towards the waves I nearly fell in. I felt like hugging that big old body of water, it had been so long. I walked along the beach to *our* lookout, where we used to sit every day for our various swims throughout the daylight hours. If some poor soul happened to be in our spot, we would squeeze in close to them until they moved. Even now I will pause as I walk by and pay homage to all the souls that loved that special place on the beach. Some were even sprinkled right there after their passing.

The weather was so divine, my friend decided to join me at the beach. We also have layers of history together in that place for near half a century now. The water called our names, and we plunged in, actually two days in a row, buoyant with joy and salt water, regardless of the cold. We visited all our cosseted spots in town and reconnected with our former customs now restored. There is little more joyful than the deprivation of pleasure that finally comes to an end and the door is open once more to another day of happiness. When the blissful two days came to an end, I swore that I would never again take my birthplace for granted. Truthfully, I never want to leave it. I'd like to see how long I could stay there until I was truly ready to leave; but so far, in my whole life, that has never happened.

My sister Rosie loved the water, same as me. She always wanted to be in it, on it, close to it. Since she lived in Turkey and I lived on the West Coast of the US, we had toyed with the idea of buying a home together in the place where we grew up, a spot where we could meet up with our friends and families and build new memories; but it wasn't to be. Maybe one day I will be able to honor our plan, but for now I find her in the water, wherever that water might be and it's a remarkably magic feeling of peace when I do. Our other sister lives on an island between England and Ireland, and she finds that same peace in her body of water in the Irish Sea and also a place where she finds our younger sister. When I returned to Turkey to visit, after Rosie passed, I found her there too. Somehow, she is in or around every body of water where I find myself. Our father was a seasoned sailor, our mother an excellent swimmer. They met in that town many years ago. Our family's sanctuary and church, if you like, has always been the water.

If you find yourself in times of trouble, in need of solace, venture forth to the place that soothes your soul. If you can't physically travel there, go there in your mind. When I was going through chemotherapy, I would travel to my birthplace in my mind. I would walk the streets; buy things I liked in the shops and spend lots of time on the beach and in the water. Randomly, I turned a corner one day away from the cottage we used to own, and my horse was tied up by the South Lookout, all saddled up and ready to go. We rode along the seafront and back via the fish shop. This all served to give me enormous comfort.

We are so lucky to live where we do, just a spit away from the Monterey Bay and all her gifts – her immense and special sanctuary, her coves and villages. There are wonderful people who live in and around the bay and love her so much. She may not be my home, but she's close to one of my homes and I will hold her close and love her all the same. The majesty of the ocean is all around us. Let us not take her for granted.

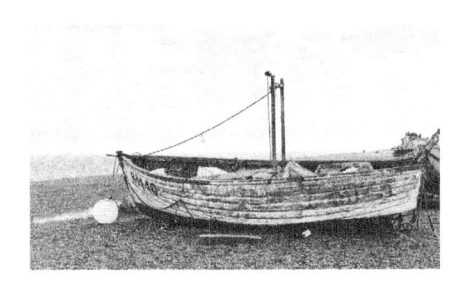

(2022)

The gammy leg

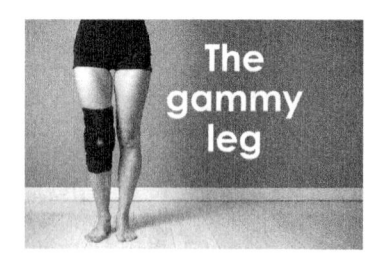

"You're limping again," he said (again.)

"YES! FULLY AWARE AGAIN OF THE FACT I'M LIMPING. DON'T MENTION IT ALL THE TIME!" (I don't think he will for a while.)

I've had a gammy leg, as father would say, for over 6 months now. When you live on a ranch, things happen all the time. Gates bang against your leg, the 50lb feed bag falls on your arm, the wire catches on your flesh. I'm a daily walking wounded ranch warrior, dripping with cuts, nicks and bruises. And I never pay attention to any of it.

Except that this time, I'm more wounded than before. My feisty mare reared in a freak way when the cow startled her, (can't make this stuff up). I had mindlessly tied her up so I could do brushing, hooves etc. Her lead rope caught, she pulled the nailed corral board out, which proceeded to whack me in the back of the leg at a rate of speed and force, knocked me to the ground (and out, I do believe) and tore up my knee pretty good. (No lectures please. I do know better….) The mare ended up at the top of the lane, towing a large piece of fence board behind her.

On that particular day, I think I walked around in shock and therefore functioned quite well. My leg was cleaned up and put in a bandage and off I went. It stiffened up badly in the afternoon and I took a nice soak in some Epsom Salts to fix me up. The next day and the following, I expected to be feeling a lot better, with all the swelling down and the wound clean. Except that is not what happened. ("Why didn't you go in to see the doctor at this point?" my friend enquired sternly.) To which I reply, who goes to the doctor when the pain is bearable, and you can still walk! We have had enough doc and hospital visits in this house – I didn't need to add myself to the list. That's what we ranch chicks do – we just get on with it.

It's almost as if I felt I deserved this gammy leg because, after all, I was going to be 60 this year. Gotta have aches and pains if you reach yet another milestone of ageing such as this! I wonder if this condition is psychosomatic, and my busy brain is just creating achy places in my head. However, the aches seemed to grow down the leg – from the knee, the accident site – to the top of the foot sometimes. I even went into the emergency room, when I was staying with my sister one time – thinking that I might have a blood clot in the leg. I didn't. It's likely muscular, the doc told me. I had sort of forgotten about my knee injury and the fact that it was still quite swollen. I put it down to fat knees and more or less investigated likely causes around the periphery of the obvious ranch accident.

My lovely doc booked me in for a bone density test and hip x-ray. Bones not too bad considering, a little osteopenia in the hip, nothing too spooky. Well, that's good news, I said to myself. I'm sure the knee will be better soon.

And then the blasted thing started to keep me awake at night, how rude. The legs were throbbing. I slapped on mineral oil, voltarol, whatever I thought might provide some relief. Aleve was on my nightstand; this had become a daily thing. ("I KNOW I'M LIMPING. DON'T EVER POINT THAT OUT AGAIN, EVER!!)

"Why didn't you go to the doctor and get a referral to an osteo?" my friend suggested again, helpfully. "I'm sure they can get to the bottom of it!" (Oh, you mean go and see a specialist that will be able to figure out my knee, leg, nerve issues? What a concept; why didn't I think of that before?) And I sort of did, but then I didn't.

The reason I have a gammy knee and a wonky leg is because I smashed it on the ground a few months back in a freak accident. The reason it is not getting better by itself is that I am basically stubborn and stupid. I have been living in complete denial these past, long 7 months and now it's time to face the music. "It might be a torn meniscus," my massage therapist noted. "You could have a torn ligament," said someone else less qualified. "You're nearly 60 – must be time for a knee replacement or two," barked someone else right at the end of the qualification line.

I called my GP and asked him when I could be seen. The first step to getting a referral and starting to fix this annoying thing is to get on the phone. "It will be a month," the receptionist said. "Okay, how about if I just see anybody, anyone at all?" "Still a month…." ('Then you people are too busy,' I said to just myself, acknowledging it was past time to change my doc office.) I made a call to another doctor and could be seen almost right away.

And here we are – about to step inside the office of a professional who will guide me towards the light in terms of starting the process of fixing my leg/knee/nerves. I'm pretty sure I shall get some flack – doctor-style – about why it took me so long to come in and how much more damage I am causing just hoping it will fix itself. But I'm ready for that. Having ignored everyone's advice and listened only to the annoying husband clacking on about my limp, I'm now to the stage when I am sick and tired of having to think about this stupid injury. I'm tired of aching and hurting and dealing with throbbing legs at night. I'm going to face this beast head on and steal back my mobility before I feel further injured or lose my sense of humor around it anymore.

When I next see you around town, I'm hoping you will notice what a good firm stride I possess, such great posture and without a single gammy leg in sight. Surely, you will then think to yourself, 'Wow, she looks good for 60!'

(2023)

The spirits of Rosie and Winston

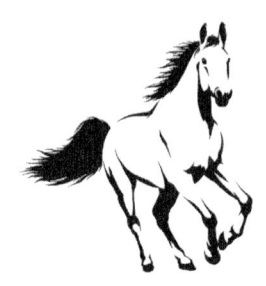

A lot of strange things happened the day the body of Sir Winston White Horse was laid to rest and his huge spirit freed. His flesh was not even cool when we were called to rescue his name-sake Winston, Jr. from Metz Road. The poor pup had been sitting there on the side of the road with a broken leg for who knows how long, watching cars drive by and leaving him behind in the dust. We picked him up – he was so sweet and grateful, despite his pain, and, as protocol requires, after a trip to the vet, he was transferred to the shelter, where he was slated for euthanasia because his leg was so badly broken and infected. We put a stop to that and immediately pulled him from the shelter as a non-profit rescue may. After about 3 months, he is now running pretty competently on all 4 legs, if a little bit inelegantly, after being used to 3 for some time. The infection has gone, and the leg was ultimately saved after a scary period, when it could have gone either way. Ultimately, wonderful vet care and love saved him.

After several potential adoptive parties reviewed his medical records and decided that his challenges were likely too much for them to handle, I had to reconcile myself to the fact that, all along, he was just waiting for me. This week, after adoption hopeful number 2 in 3 months turned him down, I decided I could not put him through any more emotional or physical stress. He would be staying forever with us at Solace, where I knew he would be safe and adored, as he should be. I knew that, if he left us, I would always worry about him and his anxiety and how he was managing elsewhere. So, the day Winston Sr. left, Winston Jr. arrived. A canine, not an equine, but a wonderful creature in his own right.

Since Winston Sr. departed this world as we know it, amazing things have happened in his place. Our three llamas – Max, Sam and Harold Malcolm Democracy – used to be quite aloof, as llamas apparently should be. Our llama shearer told us that if they became too friendly, they would be considered *maladjusted*. I never quite understood that since they never get in my physical space or threaten their humans in any way. But since Winston left, they have been roaming much less on the pasture and hanging out much more near the house with the dogs and us. When Harold would peer into the house, I'd put my arms around his long fluffy neck and we would talk about Winston and all he gave to us. We agreed that we both missed him terribly, but that we were glad we still had each other. The peering in became a daily thing, sometimes more often. He was still looking for Winston. "I think Win may have told him we would need a little more taking care of when he left," husband noted. The huge gap he would literally leave behind would need to be filled a little. And they have done that, my 3 llamas and my naughty goat; not to mention my Winston, Jr. who has kept me busy with his puppy antics and his big loving self. Though the large royal white spirit of Senior for sure still roams around Solace and I have even felt him on the breeze of a night, the llamas have helped us with our grieving and, I believe, we have helped them with theirs.

It's nearly a year since my sister passed away. Friends in Turkey have told me how many times they have seen the famous red dragonfly that has become a worldwide symbol for the spirit of Rosie. One sent me photos of the dragonfly resting on her toe by the pool. Others told me they were going to start charging pool admission, since the Rosie dragonfly had been frequenting theirs so regularly. There was never any doubt that her spirit would be mostly in Turkey, her chosen home. So far this year, I had only seen a silver blue dragonfly at home; no Rosie red ones, since the day she was transitioning from our planet to another 12 short months ago.

"You have to feel her energy, it's everywhere!" Her friend tells me. "I do," I respond. "But I want to see her dragonflies," I said, and, within minutes, there she was, flying in front of me across my secret garden. "There you are!" I exclaimed. She whooshed in and out of the pond area; then came back and rested close by. She was so close I could see her tiny eyes, mouth, nose and ears. She let me photo and video her. She tolerated my chat and my proximity for a good long while. Then she brought her flashy red boyfriend into the garden and there they played together for a while. I told everyone who would listen. I shared the photos and the video. "She came! She came after all!"

The magic made me so happy. If you are not already a believer, what I experienced might make you into one. It has been a very long and difficult year without my beautiful baby sis and my beloved Sir Winston White Horse, not to mention two of my golden oldie pups. Loss of that magnitude can take you to your knees in the worst way. But once you stand again, you might be amazed by the extent of the magic that can be found all around you. The essence of Rosie and Winston and all my beloveds are still all-around me – outside and in. Time and absence of physical presence has no bearing on love. And thank goodness for that.

(2019)

Traveling with a cold

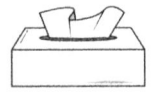

I couldn't help it, I had to cough. My throat became the most horrendous tickle fest. It was coming; everyone was looking at me. Noooo! Then, once I started, I couldn't stop. The lady near me swung around in her chair with her latte in hand and gave me the most horrid stink eye. I tried to swallow it back down; I really did. I tried to bark into the crook of my arm, but it was uncontrollable. With that came a torrent of mucus from about every orifice. I hung my head, abandoned my half-drunk tea and sloped off towards a pharmacy. This was a shameful state of affairs; I had a cold – oh and a very nasty cough. I have not had one of those since 2019 and I was not happy about it at all. Even though I am fully boostered with a flu shot for back up, I obviously could still contract a common cold with quite the flourish.

Having loaded myself up with every type of medicine supposed to stop that kind of embarrassing situation occurring again – I had tissues, cold medicine, cough syrup, cough lozenges, vapor rub and more tissues stuffed up my sleeves for back up. Surely, I could now conceal the fact that I had a cold and proceed through check-in like a normal person, albeit with a mask over my face (and you don't see many of those post pandemic-ish, despite the mega lines and too close for comfort crowds.) I was infectious and I was traveling through the airport like a criminal transporting crack cocaine. Shame on me. People have a very different attitude to others who cough and sniff these days, I noticed. Post 2020, we are all a bit precious about any noise issuing from another human that sounds something like the wretched Covid.

I should be writing an article about which cold/cough medicines work better than others, because I am here to tell you that most of our immune systems are on the floor these days, people. You too are likely to be getting a nasty contagion of some ilk, shape or form in the very near future. Lemsip is normally very winning – it's a super English cold med that I carry back to the US with me. Very soothing for the scratchy throat and dripping head – but it couldn't touch me this time. No, the mega bug that was consuming me required the big guns of Covona, that takes no prisoners. When they say it will clear your chest, they are not exaggerating. Sort of like a suction pump on steroids for the lungs.

Finally boarded onto the plane to go and see my family on the Isle of Man, I thought I had everything under control. I had had visions of them stopping me at security. 'Come this way please, madame. Ah, you WERE the one in the coffee shop who had the uncontrollable episode of exploding mucus and hacking… you had best step aside. This way, madame. Please put the bag over your head… Everyone, step to the side and let the infectious monster through!' They would lead me to quarantine in the basement of the airport, where I would not only not see my family, but I'd also miss Christmas. A lot of creative thoughts go through your head when you are high on cold medicine and crawling like a pariah through the outside world, when you know you should be tucked up in bed, watching bad tv and freely hacking to your heart's content.

The security lines at Terminal 2 were impressive. I had heard that the airport staffing levels were still an issue at London airports – as around the world indeed – and they weren't kidding. It took me an hour to shunt my way through, trying not to alert the traveling public as to my revoltingness, and yet still arrive at my chosen destination with time to spare to be able to imbibe some more cough medicine and hack up a lung.

My poor friend, who pulled her back on our trip to the coast, is nice and cozy back in her part of the world, sporting her microwave-heated strap around her injury and snuggily sipping on copious cups of tea. Why am I out here navigating this cruel universe where I am so obviously not welcome? The guy behind me on the plane was completely unsympathetic and sighed heavily every time I coughed. I even twisted my neck around at one point so he could see that I was fully masked, and he was unlikely to be receiving any of my unpopular molecules.

I made it – only an hour or so late. I thought father might not want to see me in my cold-riddled state, but like a complete trooper of the 2nd world war era (and a proud survivor of two bouts of covid in his 90's no less) he didn't seem that fussed and was nowhere near as concerned about all my unseemly noises as the airport folk. I checked in with my friends I had spent time with on the East Coast, hoping no one had contracted the same lurgy as me. They were all clear. Where on earth could I have caught it? (Trolling through the memory landmines like someone who contracted covid and couldn't place the actual site of infection or scene of the crime.) Could it have been the time I got wet feet on the beach and kept on walking? How about when I ventured forth into the cold airs with slightly damp hair? Oh, we have become so precious, haven't we. It's just a change-in-the-weather downhome common winter cold, isn't it, and I will recover, albeit with a trail of used tissues in my wake and a solid support of the very vibrant cold medicine industry.

As I awake on this beautiful day on the Isle of Man with white glistening on the grass and red-breasted robins hopping around, I'm very grateful that I feel quite well, no matter how I sound, and that, no matter what, modern medicine is here to continue to help me appear acceptable to the world outside.

If you are unlucky enough to get a cold this winter, bear in mind that a cold is no longer a cold in the eyes of the public. In their mind, you definitely have covid, RSV or something super sinister. You need to be quarantined and you'd better not be hacking over there near their personal space without at least two masks firmly positioned over all of your orifices. Consider yourself warned.

(2022)

The time for feasting

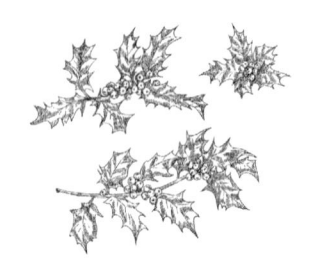

We've been on the gravy train these past couple of weeks and this train has fallen off the tracks. Going home for the holidays is not for the faint of heart, as far as the stomach and waistline are concerned. I had planned to lose 20lbs in advance of our holiday, so that I could overindulge in my home country with all the taste treats that entice this time of year and, when presented, quickly bounce back from the memory bank. I didn't lose the 20, not even a measly 10lbs in advance of our trip, even though I knew I should; but here we are, in full on beast mode. It's feasting time and everyone is talking about food and drink with fairy lights all around and twinkly trees warming up everyone's homes. I told myself I would just not eat during the daytime over the holidays, so that the evening dinner could be as opulent as I wanted. Yes, the skipping lunch or breakfast thing didn't work out either.

"Come for tea, come for dinner … have some of this lovely cake! Here's some snacks to chew on with your lovely wine appetizers…" you get the picture. It's feasting madness! Years ago, when my family was all together, we would be talking about the next meal we would be having, while we were still consuming the one on the table in front of us. Food has always been an important part of our culture and family life, but during the Christmas period it gets obscenely out of control.

It is feasting time on the East Coast of England, and I am staying in my childhood cottage by the sea. It's fish and chips for dinner – tradition on our first night at the coast – then tomorrow's dinner is out with friends in a fish restaurant – lots of wine and cream in the cooking. Don't skip dessert, why would you, it's praline profiteroles with chestnut ice cream. Try this new chestnut liqueur – it's like Christmas in a bottle. Bailey's anyone? More cheese? And the crazy thing is that the more you consume, the more you can consume. It's astounding what the human frame is capable of. I caught sight of myself sideways and was horrified. I had, in the space of 2 weeks, developed a Christmas gut.

We went out with friends to Christmas lunch at the Dolphin Pub in Thorpeness. There was soup, smoked salmon, salad, roast turkey, roast potatoes, Brussel sprouts, stuffing, gravy, bread sauce, ginger cake with sauce and cream, a bottle or two of wine … and, if you had any room left, mince pies and cream. I had walked the mile or so to the restaurant, but still. Grilled cheese and more wine for dinner and this girl is becoming positively spherical.

"Oh just a few more days of holiday," you say to yourself, as you reach for a fistful of your neighbor's French fries, or an extra gooey piece of brie that just caught your eye on the other side of the table. The day after Christmas in England is Boxing Day – the day for leftovers in most people's houses. A friend shows up with a platter of turkey, ham and trimmings, pecan pie and more. More cheese, more wine, more Christmas in a bottle.

Now we are swiftly headed towards New Year, the beginning, for many, of new and improved habits, fitness, diets and more. We, on the other hand, are headed to the island of plenty where father and sister reside, anticipating our arrival. We shall be having one lovely dinner after another, no doubt about it. "Chicken lasagna be okay for you to eat on the plane?" I ask of husband. We are, again, forward planning the food thing. I'm hoping by the time we arrive home we are both sick and tired of food and need to just quietly sip on a glass of water for a few days while we wish away our fat. I might need to get my jaws wired while I'm at it; or invest in one of those designer diet drugs that fix your excess blubber in a month.

"I'm tired of eating!" the lady tells me in the post office. "I just want to have a cup of soup and go to bed without talking to anyone, let alone cooking and cleaning up!" And the feasting season can make you feel like that. We have had so many people coming and going around our holiday house – mostly with copious amounts of food and drink – that we are actually quite tired of talking even, let alone eating. And I am definitely tired of cleaning up!

January will be much quieter in our house, that's a for sure, once we get home. We will be making soups and sipping hot tea, indulging only in early nights and reading books. The treadmill might even get a dust off, while we're at it, and I'm pondering a return to my water aerobics class when they re-open. I have had a wonderful time away in my homeland over the festive season and now my body feels absolutely disgusting!

But first we have to get through the New Year festive season with the rest of the family.... There will be full English breakfast buffets at our hotel (think bacon, eggs, sausage and so on). The seafood on the island is impressive and sister is likely to have made me a lovely, sticky ginger cake. Never mind the gins and tonics we shall likely imbibe and several glasses of very good wine, I shall just have to grin and bear it for another few days. I'll let you know how it goes.

(2023)

The year that was and the one to come

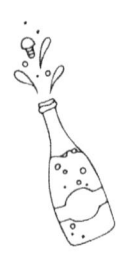

I've never been much of a fan of the *Year in Review* news magazines that are a key post in the ground at the end of each year. I don't mind recalling the good stuff; but I would not choose to go there with the grim recalls of how unpleasant human beings can be over the course of one short year. I skip through that stuff, always. It is not good for my psyche to be continuously badgering over the never-ending wrongs in the world and wishing we could all be more like dogs.

Friends of mine are fans of the *Happy Jar* – a place where you put notes about good stuff that happens throughout the year and then you revisit at the end. That's not a bad idea – at least it will make you feel like you accomplished something over the last 12 months and some of it was good. And as for New Year resolutions, I believe they belong in the trash can of good intentions. Just because I lost maybe 5lbs of the 40 I had planned for myself in the past year does not mean that a new year resolve is going to get me to my lofty goal any quicker or make me feel any better about my lack of willpower to squeeze into those jeans that I love so much – but obviously not enough to actually do anything about it.

I never was a fan of New Year – wasn't my celebration. Could have been something to do with the memory of the year that several people got crushed in Trafalgar Square and we were on the outskirts of that mele, watching the horror unfold (never went there again). Or the sadness that I still feel about my sister Rosie no longer being of this planet and the fabulous and amazing New Year celebrations I enjoyed at her home two years in a row at the end of her life. She so loved decorating for the holidays and now I like it less so. However, New Year there almost made me into a NY convert. I can so clearly recall her delight at all the American goodies and dollar bills I would schlep across the world to her home in Turkey so we could play lots of fun games with the crowds who came along to their epic parties. Fortunately, there is video and photographic evidence of these hilarious events that I sometimes watch and try not to make myself sad.

When we were young, New Year was just the long arm celebration that seemed to flow seamlessly from Christmas, since the Boxing Day feasts in our homes were a thing of epic proportions and most people had the whole week away from real life. New Year's Eve would come along, and we'd still be feasting and playing games. The trees and lights would still be up. We never seemed to tire of it. As I moved into adulthood, very often I would go to bed before midnight, unless I was on fear-watch for my critters because of the dangerous fireworks nutters like to play with. Last year there were so many people celebrating in my hometown that I swore I would never celebrate that holiday there ever again. New Year – not a thing of beauty for all folk and, as you can see from my banter, I have a very checkered relationship with it.

And here we are, the beginning of January and the house is still staggering under all the festive regalia of Christmas that came and went in a near flash. Most of my past calendars have found their way to the rubbish and recycling receptacles, my January diary is already quite well marked up and there is mud everywhere because of all the recent rains. It's a cluster. My granddaughter has just left after a muddy-rainy week with us, and we have much to clear up and reorganize before our friend from England arrives this week. And still, I need to finish clearing out the garage and unpacking boxes from our remodel. There is always much to do when I'd love to just put my feet up with a good book and think about other fun things to put in the diary. For Christmas, my daughter gave me tickets to see George Strait in Nashville this coming summer. Ooh, better organize some hotel rooms and get the structure of the trip in place – dates in the diary and all. We are going to see our son and his band play in Solvang in March – where shall we stay, never been to Solvang, how exciting. And then there's a promised trip to the Pismo coast I need to make in-between times. I had promised my friend we would have a visit in the near future, and I adore going down there, so definitely need to make that happen. My other friend and I are writing a book together about our shared childhoods – we have lots of plans to work on. I need to put together another book of my last 3 years of newspaper columns – need to squeeze that in. Oh, and work must happen at some point.

And this is how the year kicks off – with lots of plans for the future and oodles of optimism that I shall be around to enjoy it. Now if I could just get a grip on the 35lbs still left to lose, we would really be whizzing into this new year in style.

'Hello and welcome to Flight #2023. We are prepared to take off into the New Year. Please make sure your Attitude and Blessings are secured and locked in an upright position. All self-destructive devices should be turned off at this time. All negativity, hurt and discouragement should be put away….there will be NO BAGGAGE allowed on this flight. The Captain of your beautiful life has cleared us for takeoff. Have a healthy 2023 flight' – author unknown.

Waving across the valley

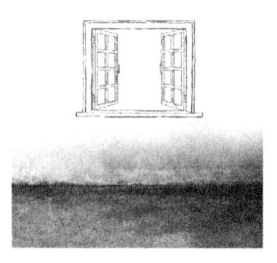

I cannot remember the first time I met her and her lovely husband. I have lived in this valley for 2 decades or more and I think it was fairly soon after I arrived - likely at a Soledad Chamber meeting, where she was an enthusiastic attendee to everything community based. Quiet and unassuming, she had a way of making you feel so very welcome in a crowd, and it didn't take long before we were the hugging kind of friends; her arms open wide with a great big smile on her face as soon as she saw me. She was a huge supporter of the Soledad Mission, and, on occasion, I'd catch her working as a volunteer in the rose garden or the gift shop. For the Mission lunches and BBQ's, she was always there, working away, the deep lines of her beautiful face as deep and furrowed as the fields around her.

She told me that she collected china teacups and saucers, and we talked about the English tradition of tea. She invited me for tea at her home and we worked hard to introduce her husband to the concept gently, because holding a delicate, bone china teacup is not something that comes exactly naturally to a rancher. We had so much fun at our tea parties, and I would take along the very best coconut macaroons for her husband's sweet tooth that he adored but was not allowed. She let me get away with it because it was me. One time I brought along her very own English china teacup and saucer from England for her lovely collection in her china cabinet, that truly delighted her. She was delighted by so many things; so very grateful and humble for all her many blessings. She always asked about my sister, during the many years when sis was ill, with heartfelt concern and she knew the agony it was for me being so very far away from her. "How's Rosie?" she would ask, her big blue eyes full of compassion. She would listen carefully and cheer me along when I stumbled.

She was a huge supporter of literacy and I remember when she and her husband Bud would volunteer at the San Vicente Elementary School. I heard about their quiet donations to local libraries and loved them even more for it. Whenever I would have a book signing, they would be there quietly supportive and loving. I know of other local authors who received the same thoughtfulness. I went to their sweet church one time in Gonzales and discovered that they were huge supporters of the food pantry next door. There were few charitable acts in our little valley that escaped their benevolence.

She told me she would look across the valley to my home and be so very glad that I lived there. She thought she could see my house from hers and that gave her comfort.

I remember standing with her in her beautiful garden and seeing the valley from her side of the street, as it were. "Gosh, Paula," I remember saying. "My view is so much better than yours!" We laughed about her living on the good side of the street with the lesser view. The Gabilans do get so very crusty brown in the summertime, yet the lush Santa Lucia Highlands stay verdant with the greens of healthy grapevines and that was her home that she loved so very much. You could not go to visit without leaving with tomatoes, or canned goods, lemons or avocadoes. Their bounty was endless.

If ever there was an example of the good side of Christianity, Paula was the perfect example. She would not thrust any beliefs down your throat or try and preach in any way; but her acts of kindness and charitable spirit alone illustrated how very pure and godly she was without trying; the essence of real Christianity. I'd call the house and get her wonderful throaty voice on the other end of the line. She had the most marvelous deep chuckle that I'm glad to be able to remember so well. She loved having her daughters around and always boasted of the love and care bestowed upon her and Bud, especially as they aged and could do less and less for themselves.

When my author friend told me of Paula's passing, I thought of her peacefully passing on to paradise within the sanctuary of her own home. For sure, there's some folk that are guaranteed a safe passage and she was one of them. She would have been surrounded by love, as she was her whole life, and, likely, tired and ready to leave her earthly body behind. She had lived a very long and, she would say, fortunate life. Her graceful spirit will be felt in the valleys around her house, certainly in the scape of bounteous fields between our homes. I looked across the valley, when I heard of her passing, and felt her looking back at me. I almost waved. I heard her delicious chuckle. Some friendships transcend.

Tales from the hammock by Paula Sarmento.

(Published some years ago in the local newspaper)

I love my hammock. Actually, it's his. I bought it for his birthday. I found it to be so comfortable in the shade under our olive trees. The breeze sometimes rocks it gently. At our age, getting into and out of it gracefully is a challenge that is not often met. He fastened a rope around a tree limb with a handle on the end to assist me in getting into and out. Well, recently I could not find the rope to assist me in getting out. I can't describe what happened. It was not a pretty sight. Old people should not rest in hammocks. I fell on his dog. Now he doesn't speak to me. Mac, not my husband.

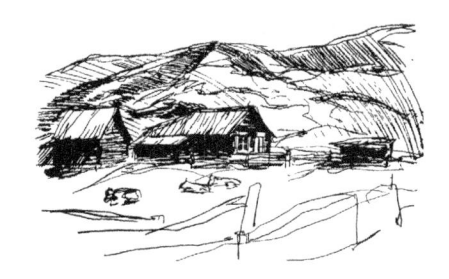

(2020)

ABOUT THE AUTHOR

Lucy Mason Jensen

Lucy was born in Aldeburgh in 1963, where she and her family spent every weekend and holiday for many wonderful years and where she still visits, whenever possible, from her home in California.

Lucy attended Friends' School Saffron Walden and then the University of London where she achieved a BA in Modern Languages. Shortly after her college days and a couple of years into her job in International Shipping in London, Lucy left the UK for the US, having become the beneficiary of a coveted green card. She lived for a few months on the East Coast and then experienced the Deep South by way of Baton Rouge, Louisiana for 2.5 years where she worked in the hotel trade.

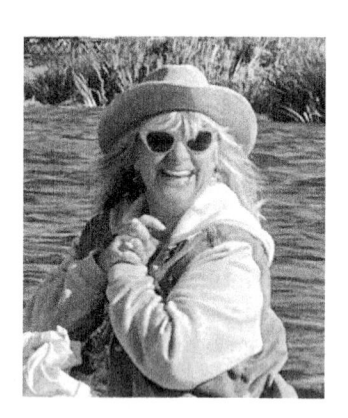

Moving to California in 1991, Lucy began work in the newspaper industry and was an employee at the Salinas Californian for 13 years and then South County Newspapers, before going into the real estate field where she currently resides. In 2003 she began writing for newspapers on a regular basis.

In 2012, Lucy published her first book, *Window on the World* – a compilation of her newspaper columns from the last several years. This was followed by *Winston Comes Home, The Animals Teach Us Everything & Other Short Tails, The Rosebud & her Brilliant Adventures, The Soup Diaries* and, most recently, her childhood story *The South Lookout – our Aldeburgh Childhoods*, which she co-authored with her childhood friend Lizzie.

Lucy began South County Animal Rescue (SCAR) in 2016 and the charity has since rescued, rehomed and transferred thousands of animals. Lucy has lived at her rescue ranch in California called Solace since 2001. She currently has 2 llamas, 1 goat, 1 pig, 1 horse, 7 dogs, about 25 cats, a bird, 2 ducks, 2 rabbits, 7 turtles, 3 chickens, 1 rooster and a baby chicken called Nugget.

lucymasonjensen@gmail.com

Printed in Great Britain
by Amazon